LANGUAGE STRATEGIES FOR OLDER STUDENTS

Vicki Prouty, M.S., CCC-SLP

Michele Fagan, M.S., CCC-SLP

Super Duper® Publications
Greenville, South Carolina

©2007 Super Duper® Publications
©2001 by Thinking Publications®
SUPER DUPER® PUBLICATIONS, a division of Super Duper®, Inc. All rights reserved. Permission is granted for the user to reproduce the material contained herein in limited form for classroom use only. Reproduction of this material for an entire school or school system is strictly prohibited. No part of this material may be reproduced (except as noted above), stored in a retrieval system, or transmitted in any form or by any means (mechanically, electronically, recording, web, etc.) without the prior written consent and approval of Super Duper® Publications.
08 07 06 05 04 03 8 7 6 5 4 3 2

Library of Congress Cataloging-in-Publication Data

Prouty, Vicki L., date.
Language strategies for older students / Vicki Prouty, Michele Fagan.
p. cm.
Includes bibliographical references.
ISBN 978-1-888222-64-7 (pbk.)
1. Speech therapy for children—Exercises. 2. Language arts—Problems, exercises, etc. 3. Children—Language—Problems, exercises, etc. 4. Language experience approach in education—Problems, exercises, etc. I. Fagan, Michele, date II. Title.

LB3454.P77 2001
371.91'4—dc21

2001027214

Printed in USA

Illustrations by Paul Modjeski

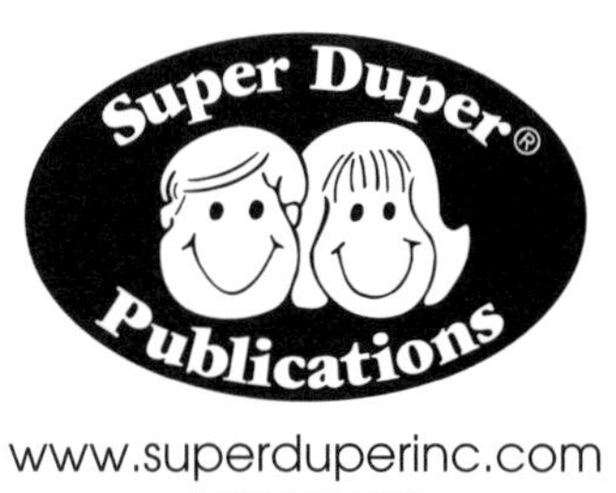

www.superduperinc.com
1-800-277-8738

To all the students, parents, and teachers
who have taught us so much

To our supportive families who cheer us on

And a special dedication to Gretchen and Walter

CONTENTS

PREFACE

Language Strategies for Older Students was developed to provide a more advanced version of the previously published books *Language Strategies for Little Ones* (1998) and *Language Strategies for Children: Keys to Classroom Success* (1997)—a version that would be appropriate for upper-elementary and middle-school grades. We wanted a program that would provide a continuum of skills starting at the kindergarten level and continuing through middle school. With the addition of *Language Strategies for Older Students,* you have a continuum of teaching ideas that use graphic strategies and literature appropriate for a preadolescent and adolescent learner. Older children will benefit from the added emphasis on written language and pragmatics, adding value and, therefore, motivation to master lesson objectives.

We have enjoyed developing this comprehensive program that has been a benefit for children and parents. We hope that educators and speech-language pathologists will find that using this resource makes them more effective and confident in meeting the needs of their students.

We extend a special thanks to the supportive administrators, teachers, parents, and students at Wells and Thomas Elementary schools in Plano, Texas. We wish to specifically thank the special education, elementary, and middle-school teachers for their input and collaboration and for allowing us to spend time in their classrooms. We also thank our reviewers—Ivy Shelton, Ellen Lamberth, Kathy Gard, and Julie Wipperfurth—whose suggestions have helped to improve this book.

INTRODUCTION

OVERVIEW

In consideration of the least restrictive environment (LRE) provision of the Individuals with Disabilities Education Act (IDEA, 1997), educators are providing services within the classroom setting when appropriate. Naremore (1995) termed this service delivery *classroom-based intervention.* Speech-language pathologists or learning disabilities specialists provide services in the classroom, sometimes teaching alongside classroom teachers and sometimes building around or supplementing the lessons being taught in the classroom (Naremore, 1995). It is as important as ever to ensure students are successful in the classroom setting—students need strategies for success. The strategies presented in *Language Strategies for Older Students* are appropriate for classroom-based intervention.

Language Strategies for Older Students is a multifaceted tool for reinforcing the communication skills of students from upper-elementary grades to middle school (grades 5–8). Two previous resources by the authors, *Language Strategies for Little Ones* (1998) and *Language Strategies for Children: Keys to Classroom Success* (1997), target language objectives for kindergarten through upper-elementary grades (K–5). *Language Strategies for Older Students* was developed to extend a continuum of language lessons by incorporating more challenging vocabulary, a written language component, and increased pragmatic communication demands.

Three units—a total of 25 lessons—focus on three primary areas: language comprehension, language expression, and story grammar knowledge. In addition, pragmatic and written language goals are embedded within each lesson. The lessons incorporate language arts concepts and other curriculum concepts as well as literature-based intervention techniques to help students develop strategies for self-prompting. *Language Strategies for Older Students* capitalizes on students' visual strengths by providing creative, visual reminders of strategies. Memorable strategy names facilitate students' internalization of the content and generalization to schoolwork, life at home, and the community. Each strategy presented in this book includes a lesson plan, *Rapid Write* application activities, and homework activities. Together, these materials maximize skill learning.

Language Strategies for Older Students is based on multiple models of learning. Hunter's (1982) lesson-cycle format and the principles of brain-based research discussed by Caine and Caine (1991) and Kavalik (1993) form the foundation of the lesson content by placing high importance on cognitive and metalinguistic skill development during language learning. In addition, *Language Strategies for Older Students* is an ideal tool for schools that are incorporating an inclusion model—all students can benefit from each strategy, but the lessons are built specifically for those students with language-learning difficulties.

The activities in the lessons appeal to students with different learning styles because they use multisensory methods (e.g., reading, writing, role-playing, and art) to promote interest and motivation and because they are relevant to students. Engaging literature is used to enhance learning and to link to classroom curriculum. The inclusion of high-interest topics (e.g., sports, environmental issues, and daily living issues) as mediums for instruction also captures students' attention because the topics are relevant to their daily lives and to their success in school.

There are many methods for implementing learning models using this resource's content. Suggestions for modifying lessons for smaller groups are included. An organizational chart (see page 15) cross-references individual lessons to communication goals.

PROGRAM GOALS

Below are the general goals targeted in *Language Strategies for Older Students* in each of the three primary areas: language comprehension, language expression, and story grammar knowledge. Pragmatic and writing goals are embedded within the three areas and in each lesson.

1. Language comprehension addresses
   - building active listening skills for all types of situations
   - discussing what can interfere (both intrinsically and extrinsically) with the listening process
   - identifying critical versus noncritical information when listening and reading
   - tuning in relevant information and tuning out irrelevant information
   - stressing evaluative listening
   - giving and receiving directions and other information
   - rereading for clarity
   - differentiating fact from opinion in a variety of contexts using evaluative thinking
2. Language expression addresses
   - identifying and switching between communication registers (i.e., social language, work/school/community language, and written language)

- recognizing and using specific language terms (e.g., subject, noun, verb, adverb, adjective)
- using precise and descriptive language (e.g., adjectives, adverbs, and synonyms) to create a more vivid message for a listener or reader
- using language skills in problem solving and higher level thinking (e.g., comparing/contrasting and identifying analogous patterns)
- understanding and using higher level vocabulary
- understanding and using figurative language (e.g., similes, idioms, and metaphors)

3. Story grammar knowledge addresses
   - using a story grammar framework for telling or retelling a story
   - applying story grammar strategies to oral and written language
   - identifying the important points in a story to develop the main idea
   - applying evaluative listening and thinking skills to link information and recognize the parts of a cause-effect relationship
   - applying in-depth and independent use of clause words
   - applying higher level inferencing skills

Each unit clearly emphasizes one of the goal areas; however, in keeping with the philosophy of whole language, all areas of communication are integrated within each unit (e.g., a lesson with a listening goal may also contain objectives with a speaking focus). The core goal areas (i.e., language comprehension, language expression, and story grammar knowledge) within *Language Strategies for Older Students* provide additional benefits to educators in the following ways:

1. To introduce an awareness of pragmatic communication and responsibilities by
   - providing activities that highlight the social importance of each strategy
   - creating a supportive environment for modeling and role-playing specific social situations
2. To integrate curriculum and language concepts by
   - emphasizing the connection between verbal and written language
   - using materials that tie in to a primary curriculum
   - planning activities that develop skills for successful communication both in and out of the school setting

3. To provide students with multisensory strategies for
   - promoting independent learning and self-prompting
   - decreasing the need for direct adult assistance
   - increasing successful experiences in an LRE
4. To develop a system that encourages parent participation by
   - increasing awareness of their child's program/goals
   - providing quick, easy, home-related activities that pertain to language goals

INTENDED USERS

Language Strategies for Older Students can be used with large groups in the classroom or in small-group settings. Educators who work to help students become independent learners in classroom, home, and community settings will find this resource useful. Strategies for learning are appropriate for all students, though the primary focus of this resource is students with language-learning difficulties. The lessons are appropriate for students in upper-elementary and middle-school grades (i.e., grades 5–8). Although most activities are intended for large or small groups, the lessons could be adapted for use with individual students.

BACKGROUND

Language Strategies for Older Students is based on sound educational models, principles, and philosophies—especially those that address the needs of a learner as a whole individual. Techniques based on these premises are embedded within the lessons and are described in the following sections.

Repeated Exposure

Caine and Caine (1991) and Kavalik (1993) described natural brain function and related implications for the teaching process. The teaching principles suggested by these researchers stress the total involvement of the brain in the emotional, physiological, and psychological learning process. In particular, they suggest that novel and challenging tasks need to be presented in connection with more familiar situations and then repeated over time. The brain's search for meaning through *patterning*—the connecting of new knowledge to prior experience—is an important component of learning.

Language Strategies for Older Students extends previously taught strategies (see *Language Strategies for Little Ones* [1998] and *Language Strategies for Children* [1997]) to an advanced level. Lessons apply strategies using more challenging vocabulary and curriculum concepts, making a direct connection to written language and including a stronger emphasis on the pragmatic components of communication. Each lesson includes a Tie-in to Prior Learning, a Focus/Relevance section, Lesson Activities, and a Closure, which summarizes the lesson concepts and provides a bridge to the next lesson.

Multisensory Methods

Rief (1993) reported that the majority of students are primarily visual learners, tactile/kinesthetic learners, or both. She cautioned educators that "only 15 percent [of students] tend to be strong auditory learners. If your teaching style emphasizes lecturing, with you doing all the talking, there is a high percentage of students you're not reaching...We need to present lessons with a combination of methods" (p. 53). The lessons in *Language Strategies for Older Students* appeal to students with different learning styles; each student has an opportunity for success. Visual learners have visual aids or graphic representations of each strategy. Clapping, physical movement, and gesturing support tactile/kinesthetic learners. Sounds, words, or rhythms engage auditory learners. Students have opportunities for practice in both large- and small-group activities. In addition, concepts from subject areas (e.g., math, science, and social studies) can be integrated into lessons to draw on students' academic strengths.

Strategy-Based Intervention

Cognitive strategies (e.g., analyzing) and metacognitive strategies (e.g., planning and organizing) are important for effective language learning (Oxford, 1994). There should be plenty of opportunity for practicing strategies during a language lesson. When teaching strategies, educators should include explanations, handouts, activities, and home practice materials (Oxford). *Language Strategies for Older Students* is a strategy-based program. Each strategy has an accompanying visual graphic, an activity for learning it, and an opportunity for demonstrating use of the strategy both orally and in written form. The strategies require students to self-evaluate and self-monitor their communication beyond the classroom setting, such as in the community in social situations (e.g., when talking with friends) or at school (e.g., when listening to a teacher or working on class projects within a group). In addition, the strategies provide a plan for repairing interactions when breakdowns occur for those learners who find vocabulary or concepts in classroom curricula challenging.

Whole Language Philosophy

Whole language has been described as a partnership between intent and learning, focusing on meaning and relevance as the catalyst for learning (Wagner, 1989). Whole language capitalizes on the social aspects of communication because the philosophy encourages teachers to keep language whole and involve children in using it to meet children's needs (Genishi, 1988; Goodman, 1986). While the whole language philosophy is not applied in its purest form in *Language Strategies for Older Students,* language learning is addressed in context, as it occurs, in language rich situations. Lessons integrate listening, speaking, reading, and writing at a level appropriate to students' needs.

Curriculum-Based Intervention

Intervention that integrates curriculum vocabulary and concepts with communication goals is termed *curriculum-based intervention* (A. Bird, personal communication, September 1, 1992). This approach to intervention creates a relevant context for language learning. *Language Strategies for Older Students* is curriculum-based. It is important to remember that curriculum-based and classroom-based intervention emphasize communication goals, not curriculum content, but use curricular concepts as the stimuli for improving communication. Since each school district has its own curricular goals, activities should be adapted to include relevant curriculum goals and objectives.

Literature-Based Intervention

Lessons in *Language Strategies for Older Students* embed high-interest, engaging, and entertaining literature that can be used to learn language and can be linked to classroom concepts. For example, *Turn of the Century* by Ellen Jackson (1998) is used to emphasize comparing and contrasting. The book provides historical information from the perspective of children living at 100-year intervals between the years 1000 and 2000. The clever combination of fact and fiction engages students and adults and creates excellent opportunities for comparing and contrasting while also connecting to curriculum concepts (e.g., map skills or history). The literature used in *Language Strategies for Older Students* is listed in the Bibliography (see page 177).

Connection to Written Language

Since many students, particularly those who have reading or writing difficulties, are visual learners, tactile/kinesthetic learners, or both (Rief, 1993), they may actively avoid tasks related to written language. However, *Language Strategies for Older Students* teaches writing in a pragmatic context;

students learn that sometimes the purpose of writing is formal (e.g., when writing a report, a letter, or a textbook) and other times it is informal (e.g., when serving as a memory device for assignments or when writing a message to oneself) and spelling, penmanship, and other standards of accuracy are not as important. Opportunities for using written language formally, informally, or both are provided in every lesson.

The connection between oral and written language is also reinforced through short, written activities called *Rapid Writes.* Research has shown that building fluency in writing does not require completing a writing process (e.g., outlining, prewriting, editing, and publishing) for each assignment (Chadwell, 1994). Short, focused assignments where two or three specific criteria are focused on (e.g., writing three sentences with an adjective or adverb included in each sentence and using correct punctuation) can build fluency and confidence because the structure is defined and students perceive the task as manageable. This philosophy is coupled with a method from the Treatment and Education of Autistic and Related Communication Handicapped Children (TEACCH) approach for students with autism (Mesibov, Adams, and Klinger, 1998) and forms the basis of writing assignments in *Language Strategies for Older Students. Rapid Writes*—short written activities—allow students to immediately apply new strategies learned to writing.

Pragmatic Activities

Paul (1995) defined *pragmatics* as the use of language in a communicative context. Because upper-elementary and middle-school students experience the social challenges of preadolescence, emphasis is placed on applying each strategy to home, school, and community situations. Furthermore, each new strategy builds on previous strategies learned, and students develop a new understanding of communication dynamics in various situations. *Language Strategies for Older Students* is rich with opportunities for using new skills in pragmatically appropriate ways.

Hunter's (1982) Lesson Model

Hunter's (1982) lesson-cycle format reinforces the principles of brain-based research by providing repeated exposure to a concept within a lesson. The lesson format used in *Language Strategies for Older Students* is an adaptation of Hunter's model. Hunter presents the following lesson components that maximize student learning:

1. *Objectives*—describe the desired change in student behavior
2. *Anticipatory Set*—sets the stage for learning by sparking student interest and curiosity about the lesson

3. *Modeling*—presents examples of behaviors an educator wants students to perform independently
4. *Guided Practice*—checks students' level of understanding of the concept before moving on
5. *Independent Practice*—provides tasks to be completed until students show mastery of the lesson concepts or skills

These components are embedded in all *Language Strategies for Older Students* lessons. They are further explained in the next section.

UNIT COMPONENTS

Goal Setting

Language Strategies for Older Students stresses responsibility for communication and ownership of communication goals. For each of the three units, students write goals with educator help and form their own plans for improvement. Students think about when the goals are relevant at home, at school, and in the community and write their thoughts on their goal sheets. Before beginning a new unit (or in the case of Unit Three, at the end of the unit), students revisit their previously completed goal sheets and discuss their progress in achieving the goal and application examples.

The goal sheets are taken home, so students can share their goals with family members. While students will develop skills at school, some of the practice must occur at home, so students can generalize learning into other situations. Goal sheets serve as documentation of progress and help communicate progress to family members. Students are encouraged to have their goal sheets initialed by a family member and returned to school. Goal setting is an extremely successful and motivational teaching strategy. Students feel informed about their progress, which may help them become more enthusiastic and motivated; this progress is demonstrated by a change in students' attitudes and performance.

Lessons

Every lesson includes the following teaching components:

1. *Objectives*—clearly state the change expected in student behavior within each lesson, though measurable elements should be added based on each individual's needs.
2. *Introduction*—parallels the anticipatory set of Hunter's (1982) model. It has two elements: Tie-in to Prior Learning and Focus/Relevance. The Tie-in to Prior Learning is a review of the previous lesson (if appropriate). It sets the stage for connecting prior experience with new knowledge. The Focus/Relevance element establishes an anticipatory set, resulting in a more

meaningful entry into a topic. Focusing techniques include posing a provocative question or a statement of the objective. The purpose of this component is to have students clear their mind of irrelevant ideas and get ready to learn.

3. *Lesson Activities*—present the basic information necessary to meet the objectives. Modeling a strategy or process is essential to ensure understanding. Hunter (1982) stressed the use of keywords and simple diagrams in a lesson, and these techniques comprise the language strategies presented. Each lesson activity includes checking for understanding via signalled answers or a sampling of individual responses (either oral or written).

4. *Closure*—includes a discussion of lesson relevance and value to promote transfer of learning and guided practice. *Teaching for transfer,* as Hunter (1982) called it, involves making the information meaningful by connecting past and future knowledge to present learning. The educator identifies critical parts of the present learning and ties them to students' lives using facilitative techniques such as mnemonics or memory helpers. *Teaching for meaning* (i.e., introducing short meaningful chunks of information for students to practice), as Hunter termed it, is included through guided and independent practice. Lessons also apply Hunter's principle of *distributed practice* in that strategies previously taught are revisited periodically as they apply to a current lesson. This helps to improve retention of the strategy.

Strategy Graphics

Each lesson has one full-page graphic that serves as a visual aid to help students remember the strategy. This graphic should be duplicated and enlarged to create a poster, which can be colored and laminated for durability. The poster should be placed on a classroom wall or bulletin board and referred to while students are learning the strategy or when the strategy is reviewed. The graphic can also be used to create transparencies for overhead projectors to use while teaching the lesson.

Rapid Writes

The connection between oral and written language is also reinforced through short written activities or *Rapid Writes* found in each lesson. *Rapid Writes* present structure for completing assignments by asking four critical decision-making questions: (1) What is my job? (2) What will I need to complete the job? (3) How will I know when I'm finished? (4) What will I do when I'm finished? The answers to these questions are listed as guiding statements in a shaded box for each *Rapid Write*. Following initial instruction, students can work independently and develop skill in using written information (e.g., text, pictures, and specific examples) to complete an assignment. When students request help, the educator should take a nonverbal approach and point to the steps in the shaded box on the *Rapid Write*, encouraging students to reread for clarity, check their own progress, and look to the next step listed. This approach benefits those with language-processing difficulties by helping them become more efficient workers and value text as a helpful tool.

Rapid Writes can be adapted for varying reading levels. For example, Rebus symbols can be added to facilitate reading. The brief *Rapid Write* assignments allow students to apply a strategy to writing immediately following lesson activities.

Just Do It!

At least one *Just Do It!* review activity is provided for each unit, so students can share and practice the targeted skills with their families. Each *Just Do It!* includes strategy vocabulary and stresses key points that students might apply to tasks in the home or community environment. If students complete this activity, family members are asked to sign the sheet and return it to school by a set date. Establishing a reward system for completing the activity and returning signed sheets helps to ensure this important step is done.

The *Just Do It!* review activities encourage family-child involvement and give family members examples of how home practice can support communication skills in an easy and useful way. Students learn that their parents value good communication skills.

PROCEDURES FOR USE

Language Strategies for Older Students is written with a flexible format, so educators can develop communication intervention lessons using their own teaching style. At the same time, much of the lesson material is specifically written to model direct-instruction procedures. It provides a framework that a beginning professional can follow or one that an experienced educator can incorporate into a previously existing program. The units and lessons will spur new ideas.

Presenting the Lesson

Each lesson is presented for use in a classroom setting. Most lessons can be taught within a 30-minute class period. However, lessons can be extended over several class periods to ensure understanding or to give students more opportunities to practice a new strategy. Lessons with more than one activity may require more than one session to complete.

Lessons were written for upper-elementary and middle-school students. Expand and modify the content within each lesson to fit different levels of student ability. Hints and notes are included in many of the lessons to provide helpful information or suggestions for adapting the lessons in different ways. The hints also facilitate the flow of the lesson and are provided to help prevent potential problems.

Although the lessons are intended for use in a classroom setting, they are easily adapted for smaller groups by allowing more individual responses and participation. Using the lessons within a small-group setting allows you to spend whatever time is necessary to ensure that all students have an understanding of the targeted objectives. A small-group setting also provides more opportunities for independent practice.

Higher level questioning can extend any lesson; Bloom's (1956) taxonomy lists a hierarchy of questioning beginning at the knowledge level, where only content questions are asked (e.g., "What was the name of the main character?" and "Who was at the party?"). More difficult questions can be asked that require students to manipulate information, arrive at conclusions, or draw inferences (e.g., "Why did John decide to leave?" "Do you think he made a good choice?" "Why or why not?" and "What else could he have chosen to do?").

Suggestions for using literature are included whenever a piece of literature is used with the lesson. When using literature, the author, illustrator, book cover, and any relevant vocabulary should be discussed. Note particular components of the book (e.g., a figurative language expression or words with multiple meanings) while reading the story rather than discussing them out of context before reading the story. Lessons including literature describe literary highlights specific to the particular story listed in the Materials section of the lesson. Suggestions for literature use and discussion are provided before reading, during reading, and/or after reading. If the book suggested is not available in your setting, another similar book can be substituted. If substituting another book, adapt the lessons as appropriate.

Before beginning any lesson, gather the necessary materials. Create the strategy poster using the graphic provided. The poster is a visual cue to help students remember the strategy. It is an integral part of the lesson and can be referred to in subsequent lessons. Duplicate and enlarge the graphic, color it if desired, mount it onto construction paper or poster board, and laminate it for durability if desired. You could also make an overhead transparency of the graphic for writing and erasing words easily. Sometimes a lesson requires writing information where all students can see it. A chalkboard and chalk could be used as the media for writing the information, but a dry erase board or an overhead projector and markers work just as well. If co-teaching with a classroom teacher in the regular education setting or in a resource-room setting, give a copy of the poster to the classroom teacher or post it somewhere in the room, encouraging the teacher and students to carryover the strategies to other lessons.

Certain parts of the lessons have been scripted to give you an example of presenting the idea. The scripts are only examples and should be reworded to fit your teaching style and students' learning needs.

The scripts, for example, in the Focus/Relevance section of the lessons are intended to lure students into a lesson, so they are curious, excited, ready to problem solve, and immediately engaged in the lesson. However, you may choose a more direct focus by simply stating the purpose of the lesson for students.

Just Do It! review activity sheets are provided, so students can share and complete the targeted strategies and skills with their family members. The activities generally ask students to summarize the strategy and apply it to a home situation (e.g., listening for critical information when baby-sitting) or community situation (e.g., listening for directions to a friend's house). This encourages family-child involvement and gives family members examples of how home practice can support communication skills in a quick, easy way.

Additional Techniques

The following techniques, occasionally mentioned within the lessons, are useful methods for teaching in an inclusive classroom. To ensure the participation of all students when in a large group and to keep students engaged during an activity or a brief discussion portion of a lesson, employ a variety of these techniques:

- *Golf clap*—involves tapping the first two fingers on the palm of the opposite hand. This noiseless clap can be used by an entire class to show understanding of a concept (e.g., when one student has been called on to give an answer, other students can indicate that they were thinking of the same answer by using the golf clap). Keep more students engaged by acknowledging those students signaling identical responses with their golf clap (e.g., "I see that John and Sara were thinking the same answer as Tom"). Extend responses by asking for different answers or ideas.
- *Signaling*—shows agreement or disagreement with a concept through signals (e.g., showing thumbs-up or thumbs-down, flash cards, marking a response on a dry erase board, or raising hands). Decide with students what the signal will be.
- *Brainstorming*—involves having students generate as many ideas as possible. Ideas are not judged as appropriate or inappropriate when brainstorming, because implausible responses can generate new alternatives.
- *Choral response*—incorporates responses done in unison as a large group. This can be done while answering questions or to complete a cloze procedure sentence.
- *Whisper voices*—minimizes any disruption or disturbance of nearby classrooms when an entire class is responding in unison in a choral response.

- *Six-inch voices*—provide a way to describe the volume students should use when working in small groups or pairs. Six-inch voices are voices that can only be heard six inches away. This technique helps to keep the volume level in the classroom manageable.
- *Learning groups*—encourage maximum student participation through small-group work. If you are versed in the principles of cooperative learning as described by Johnson, Johnson, and Johnson Holubec (1990), these principles can be applied. When working in small groups, one student could act as a recorder and another as a reporter. The recorder writes or marks in some way the group's ideas and the reporter shares the ideas with the large group. These roles can be assigned by saying something like "Today the students wearing the most blue will be the recorders and the students wearing the most brown will be the reporters." The learning group strategy gives all group members the opportunity to participate in each role.
- *Role-playing activities*—allow students to practice communicating in social situations, such as asking for directions, within a safe and structured environment.

CROSS-REFERENCE CHART

The cross-reference chart on page 15 provides a cross-reference of units/lessons and communication goals. The chart marks the goals targeted directly within each lesson with an X. The chart also indicates goals that are indirectly targeted within each lesson with a dot. Use this cross-reference to develop goals and objectives for students' individualized education programs (IEPs) if desired. To use objectives for IEPs, measurable components should be added.

Cross-Reference Chart

GOALS — UNITS/LESSONS	UNIT 1	Critical Information	Static	Hit the Bull's-Eye	Fact and Opinion	UNIT 2	Code-Switching Tools (Comm. Registers)	Code-Switching Tools (Subject/Verb)	Code-Switching Tools (Adverb/Adj.)	Code-Switching Tools (Synonyms)	Word Power	Discover the Pattern	Smooth Sailing	Ultimate Word Power Tools	Extreme Communication	UNIT 3	Story Formula	Main Idea	The Detail Trail
Identify Critical vs. Noncritical		X	•	•	•								•					•	
Tune In Relevant/ Tune Out Irrelevant Info		•	X	•	•		•	•	•	•	•	•	•	•	•		•	•	•
Give/Receive Directions		•	•	X	•		•	•	•	•	•	•	•	•	•		•	•	•
Differentiate Fact/Opinion					X														
Identify/Switch Communication Registers				•			X	•	•	•									
Recognize/Use Subjects/Verbs								X	•	•			•	•	•				
Recognize/Use Adverbs/Adjectives									X				•	•	•				
Recognize/Use Synonyms			•				•			X		•	•	•					•
Compare/Contrast Items		•	•	•	•		•	•	•	•	X	•	•	•	•		•	•	•
Recognize Word Relationships												X	•	•					•
Define Words		•	•	•	•		•	•	•	•	•	•	X	•	•		•		•
Understand/Use Figurative Language			•				•			•				X	X		•		
Identify/Use Story Grammar Elements																	X		
Identify Details/Main Idea																	•	X	X
Recognize Cause/Effect																	•		X

X = Targeted goal

• = Additional goal that is reinforced

UNIT ONE

GOAL-SETTING ACTIVITY ONE

GOAL

To encourage self-improvement through goal setting

BACKGROUND INFORMATION

The purpose of this lesson is to help students learn the steps for setting and meeting a goal (i.e., identifying a need, formulating a goal, practicing the steps to reach the goal, revising a goal as needed, and evaluating progress) and apply the steps to setting a goal for listening. Rather than expecting students to set goals independently, the goal-setting process is modeled. Writing a goal for listening could be teacher directed, but reflection on the need for the goal and how the goal might be useful will be individual for each student since each student's use of the goal is different. Note that Unit One has a mix of goals, not all of which involve listening. However, effective listening forms the basis of success for lessons in this unit, so this goal-setting activity will focus on improving listening skills.

OBJECTIVES

1. Understand the following vocabulary terms: *goal, skills,* and *achieve.*
2. Become aware of the importance of practicing specific listening skills in a variety of settings.
3. Write a goal related to listening and identify when this skill is important at home, at school, and in the community.

MATERIAL

1. *Goal Setting: Activity One* (See page 22; duplicate one per student.)

INTRODUCTION

Tie-in to Prior Learning

Discuss with students the idea that when we learn to do something new it can be hard at first but gets easier with practice. Elicit tasks that require a number of steps to practice, such as scoring a soccer goal or playing a musical instrument. Relate these tasks to setting, practicing, and achieving a goal that requires learning several skills (e.g., throwing, catching, or hitting a ball to become a better baseball player).

Focus/Relevance

1. Ask students to tell what they know about listening. Allow time for students to respond and discuss briefly. Tell students that they may be thinking about listening in a different way in this unit.
2. Tell students that learning is easier when goals are set and steps for achieving them are planned. Achieving a goal may require a strategy—a standard way of attacking a problem. Setting a goal and practicing the steps to reach the goal can help students achieve and accomplish many different skills at home, at school, and in the community.

LESSON ACTIVITIES

1. Give each student a copy of *Goal Setting: Activity One*. Write the word *listening* where everyone can see it. Ask if students think effective listening is an easy goal to achieve. Ask students if they have ever missed a homework assignment, missed items on a test, or missed out on something important that the teacher said even though they heard the teacher say it. Explain that there are several skills involved in being an effective listener just as there are several skills involved with being a good baseball player. Explain that just as a baseball player needs to concentrate and practice the skills needed to improve, students need to identify the listening skills they could improve.
2. Discuss situations in which students feel that they could be better listeners at school, at home, and in the community. Students might think of situations, such as paying closer attention in class, not becoming distracted, or following a coach's directions. Tell students that one of their main goals during this unit is to become effective listeners at home, at school, and in the community. Write this goal where everyone can see it. Tell students that to be effective means that they are listening to hear critical and relevant information and they will learn more about how to be effective listeners in the lessons to follow.
3. Read through *Goal Setting: Activity One* as a group and check for understanding. Have students complete the goal statement on their goal sheets by adding the word *effective.* Tell students to write down examples of situations when they need to be effective listeners at home, at school, and in the community. Discuss their responses.

HINT: If students have difficulty generating situations, use one of the following ideas.

An example of when this goal is important

- at home is when my parents give instructions for using something
- at school is when the teacher gives an assignment
- in the community is when my friend tells me the date of her party

CLOSURE

Summarize the lesson, review its relevance to students, and tie it to future learning. Recap for students by explaining that they have set an important goal and in the next lesson they will begin working on the first step to achieve their goal. Have them sign and date *Goal Setting: Activity One.* By signing and dating the goal sheet, they are promising to concentrate and work on the goal. Explain that you will also sign their goal sheets as a promise to help each student reach his or her goal. Encourage students to take the goal sheet home to share with their family, but request that they return it by a set time with a family member's initials. Keep the goal sheets for future reference as they will be used again during the next goal-setting lesson *(Goal-Setting Activity Two).* When the goal sheets are returned, you might want to keep them all in one folder or create a separate folder for each student.

HINT: Offer a tangible or social reward for returning the goal sheet with a family member's initials.

GOAL SETTING

ACTIVITY ONE

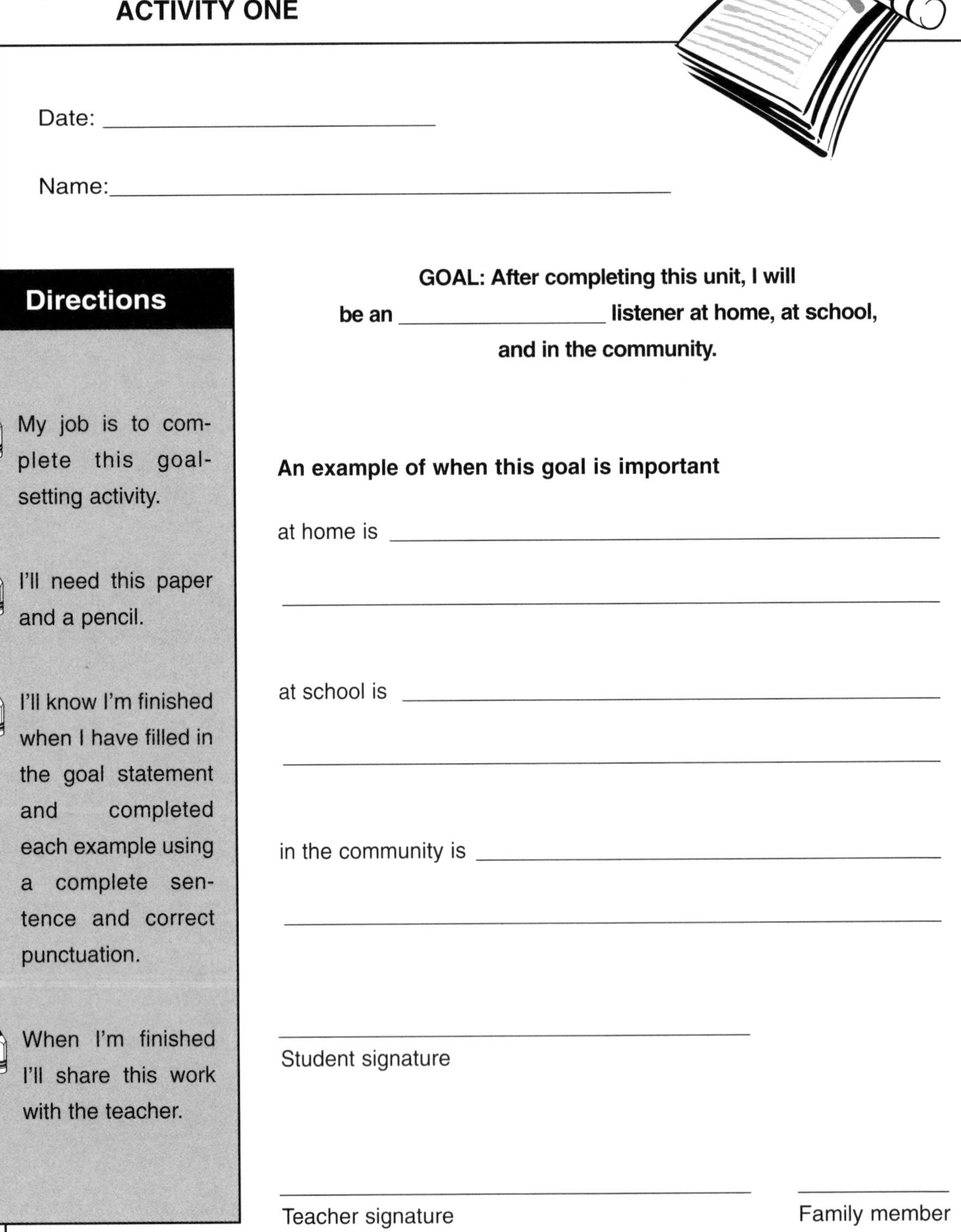

Date: ____________________

Name: ______________________________

Directions

- My job is to complete this goal-setting activity.
- I'll need this paper and a pencil.
- I'll know I'm finished when I have filled in the goal statement and completed each example using a complete sentence and correct punctuation.
- When I'm finished I'll share this work with the teacher.

GOAL: After completing this unit, I will be an ____________ listener at home, at school, and in the community.

An example of when this goal is important

at home is ______________________________

____

at school is ______________________________

____

in the community is ______________________________

____

____
Student signature

____
Teacher signature

____
Family member initials

© 2001 *Thinking Publications.* Duplication permitted for educational use only.

CRITICAL INFORMATION: IDENTIFYING SIGNALS (PART I)

GOAL

To identify critical versus noncritical information

BACKGROUND INFORMATION

The purpose of this lesson is to help students identify the cues that signal critical information in the classroom. For example, a teacher often uses signaling phrases, such as "I hope you are listening carefully" or "You may see this information again." Textbooks also provide valuable clues for identifying critical information, such as use of bold or italic print and shadow boxes for important information. Once students have been introduced to critical information in classroom activities *(Part I)*, they will extend that knowledge to home and community situations *(Part II)*.

OBJECTIVES

1. Understand the terms *critical* and *noncritical*.
2. Identify spoken and written cues at school that signal important information.

MATERIALS

1. *Identifying Signals* graphic (See page 26; duplicate and enlarge the graphic, color it, mount it onto construction paper or poster board, and laminate it for durability if desired.)
2. Textbook (Use any science or social studies textbook to show how important information is highlighted or set apart.)
3. *Critical Sentence Strips* (See pages 27–28; duplicate and enlarge the sentence strips, laminate for durability if desired, and cut into strips.)
4. *Rapid Write: Critical Information (Part I)* (See page 29; duplicate one per student.)

INTRODUCTION

Tie-in to Prior Learning

Remind students that in *Goal-Setting Activity One* they set goals that would help them be effective listeners. Discuss the difference between this school year and last. Ask if they think this year is harder than last year and discuss why. Tell students that once again they will be exploring ways to make this their most successful year in school. Remind them that it always takes practice to get better when learning new or harder skills.

Focus/Relevance

1. Tell students to turn to their neighbor and give him or her five. After they have responded in some way, congratulate them on following the two critical parts of your direction by turning to a neighbor and exhibiting some type of interaction. Comment on the different ways they interacted (e.g., some students might have slapped hands high and others slapped hands low).

2. Discuss the five listening components (i.e., no talking, hands free of objects, listening to the speaker, eyes on the speaker, and sitting still). Remind students that when they were younger, using the five components may have been how they learned to listen. They will continue to use these five components to be effective listeners, but now they will learn other strategies.

LESSON ACTIVITIES

1. Show the *Identifying Signals* poster and discuss the message that a traffic light sends to drivers. A green light signals a driver to proceed through the intersection, a yellow light signals a driver to slow down and prepare to stop, and a red light signals a driver to come to a complete stop. Tell students that they must also be aware of signals at home and in school. Point out that they should be listening for signals the teacher gives or signals in a book that indicate get ready to slow down, stop, and "Take action! Write it down!" Explain to students that *critical information* means important information.

2. Discuss comments about this school year that were mentioned at the beginning of the lesson. Stress that students can be more successful in school by practicing the skills that their teachers already expect them to know (e.g., finding important information in a textbook or knowing when a teacher has given an important fact or direction). Ask students how they know when a teacher has said something really important that they will need to remember. Brainstorm teacher comments, such as "This is really important" or "If I were you, I'd write this down." Write the ideas where everyone can see them. Ask if their teachers ever talk about things that are not important or not critical to know. Brainstorm examples, such as when a teacher drifts off to talk about a hobby. Stress that when students have identified information that is critical, they will want to remember it and may want to write it down. Summarize that listening and reading for critical information means looking for important information.

3. Ask students if a writer can signal critical information in a textbook. Show students several sample textbooks, such as science and social studies textbooks, or a novel they have read in class. Discuss and demonstrate how writers visually indicate critical versus noncritical information by using bold or italic print or increasing the size of the print for chapter headings.

Have students flip through the textbook or novel and identify other things that get their attention. Model summarizing a chapter by selecting a book and saying, for example:

> *This chapter seems so long and has lots of pages, but when you find the important or critical information, you may need to know only two or three critical ideas. In this chapter on the solar system, you will learn about the nine planets and how their distance from the sun effects their environment.*

Point out any visual or graphic signals within the text that indicate critical information. Refer students to the *Identifying Signals* poster. Point out the examples of critical signals that a textbook might have that alert students to "Take Action! Write it down!"

4. Tell students that they will now read sentence strips and decide if the information is critical. Place the *Critical Sentence Strips* in the center of a table, and have students take turns choosing a strip and then reading it. To keep all students actively involved in this activity, have the whole group signal whether they think the information is critical or noncritical with a thumbs-up or thumbs-down. Discuss responses after each turn. Note that there is no one correct response; context is important in determining whether a sentence is critical or noncritical. For example, the sentence "Your friend discusses her pet" could be considered noncritical if two friends are just chatting but critical if the pet is sick and you are pet sitting for your friend and need special instructions to care for the animal. Tell students that when they signal that information is critical they should remember that it means "Take action! Write it down!" Noncritical information is not important for the moment.

5. Hand out *Rapid Write: Critical Information (Part I)*. Read through the directions as a group and check for understanding. Give students time to list three examples of critical signals they might hear a teacher give and three examples of critical signals they might see in textbooks. Then have students write two examples of when they might hear critical information at school and two possible consequences for missing critical information. Discuss their different responses.

CLOSURE

Summarize the lesson, review its relevance to students, and tie it to future learning. Tell students to summarize the two kinds of information they must be able to differentiate in the classroom or in their textbooks. Elicit the terms *critical* and *noncritical.* Challenge students to remember examples of both critical and noncritical information to share in the next lesson. In the next lesson *(Critical Information: Identifying Signals [Part II])*, they will be learning how effective listening can help make them better friends and more successful at home.

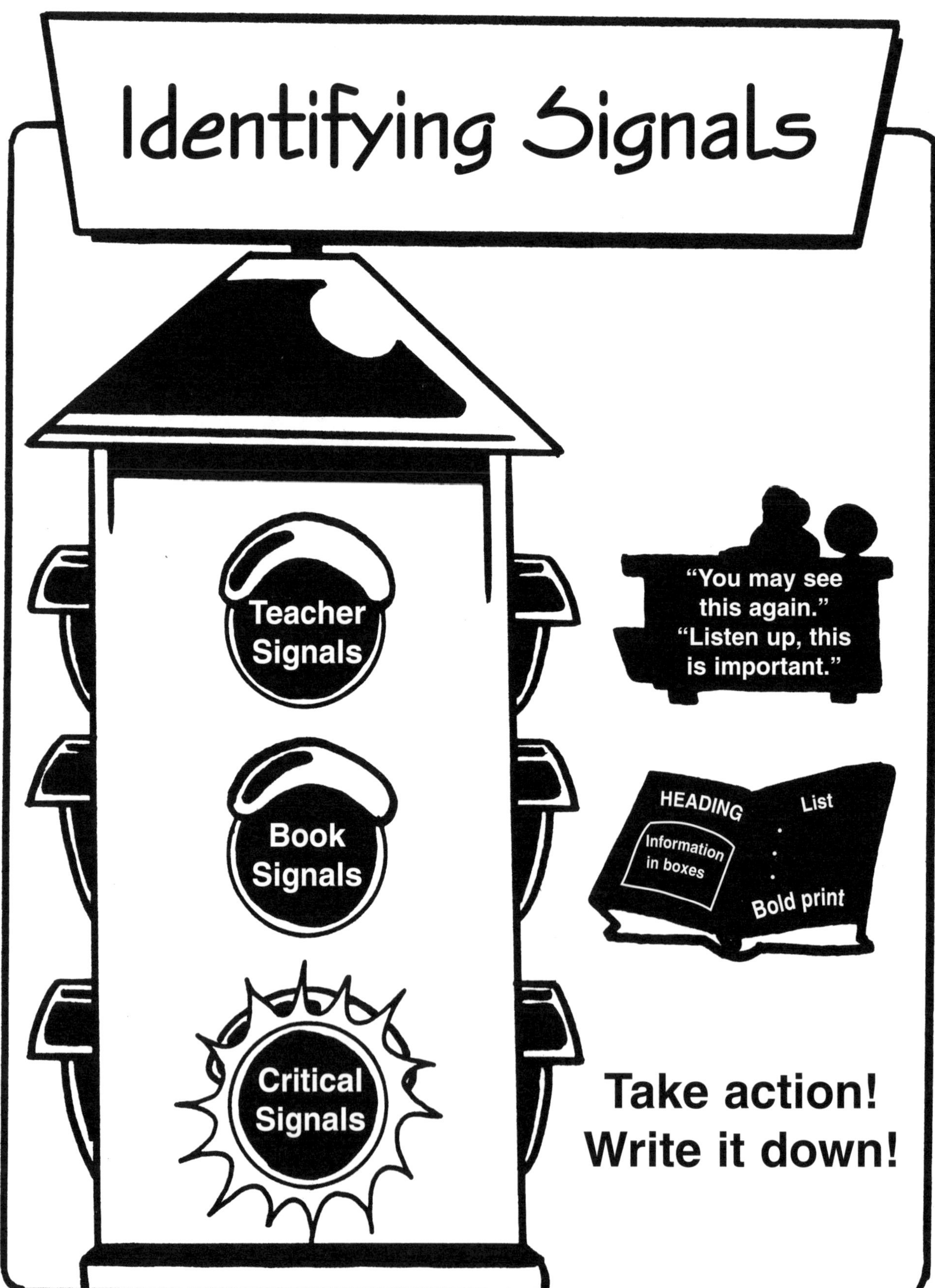

© 2001 *Thinking Publications.* Duplication permitted for educational use only.

Critical Sentence Strips

You are getting directions to a friend's house.

Your friend tells you the date of his party.

Your teacher states the chapter to read for homework.

The principal announces the time and date of the school open house.

The dentist calls to leave a message about your dad's dentist appointment.

You see bold headings in a chapter in your science book.

Your friend tells you the movie times.

Your coach gives directions for a play to the team.

Your teacher says, "You may be seeing this again."

The student council poster tells the date and time for the dance committee meeting.

© 2001 *Thinking Publications.* Duplication permitted for educational use only.

Your teacher says she enjoyed meeting your parents.

Your teacher talks about her visit to an art museum.

Your friend discusses her pet.

Your friend shares something funny that happened at a party.

Your sister tells you what she will wear to a party.

Your coach tells about her greatest sports moment.

Your teacher describes why he liked a chapter in a book he read.

You read a comic book and there are no headings.

Your brother shares details about the two movies he just saw.

Your coach says, “Play hard and do your best!”

© 2001 *Thinking Publications.* Duplication permitted for educational use only.

Rapid Write

CRITICAL INFORMATION (PART I)

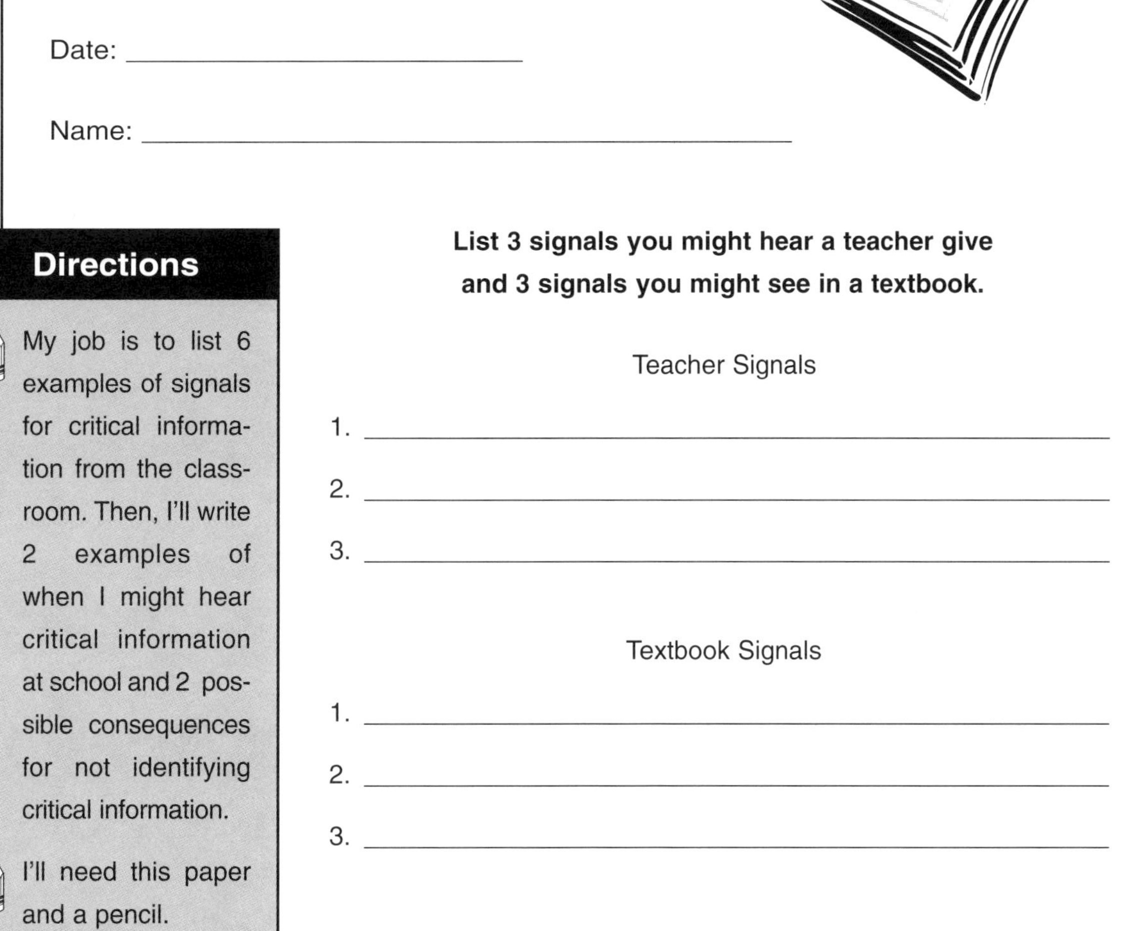

Date: ____________________________

Name: ____

Directions

- My job is to list 6 examples of signals for critical information from the classroom. Then, I'll write 2 examples of when I might hear critical information at school and 2 possible consequences for not identifying critical information.
- I'll need this paper and a pencil.
- I'll know I'm finshed when I have listed 6 signals and written 4 complete sentences.
- When I'm finished I'll share this work with the teacher.

List 3 signals you might hear a teacher give and 3 signals you might see in a textbook.

Teacher Signals

1. ____
2. ____
3. ____

Textbook Signals

1. ____
2. ____
3. ____

Complete these sentences.

I might hear critical information at school when:

1. ____
2. ____

If I miss critical information, these are possible consequences:

1. ____
2. ____

© 2001 *Thinking Publications.* Duplication permitted for educational use only.

CRITICAL INFORMATION: IDENTIFYING SIGNALS (PART II)

GOAL

To identify critical versus noncritical information

BACKGROUND INFORMATION

The purpose of this lesson is to help students identify the cues that signal critical information at home or in the community. As in *Part I* of this unit where a teacher uses signaling phrases, friends and family also use signaling phrases, such as "I hope you remember that…" or "This is really important to me," to signal critical information. This lesson addresses signals at home or in the community.

OBJECTIVES

1. Listen to a peer to identify critical information about him or her.
2. Relate critical information about oneself in a group setting.

MATERIALS

1. *Identifying Signals* poster (Created earlier)
2. Small ball or object (See step 1 under Lesson Activities.)
3. *Rapid Write: Critical Information (Part II)* (See page 32; duplicate one per student.)

INTRODUCTION

Tie-in to Prior Learning

Remind students that in the last lesson (*Critical Information: Identifying Signals [Part I]*) they identified the signals that a teacher or a textbook might use to indicate important information and had to evaluate different situations to determine if critical information was being given or shown. Remind students that identifying critical information will keep them focused on what is really important for them to know or remember rather than having to remember a lot of unimportant details. When they find out what is really important to remember, they should "Take action! Write it down!"

Focus/Relevance

Ask students if they have ever tried to tell a friend or family member about something exciting that happened but the listener started talking about something else and never really heard them. Ask how that made them feel and whether they have ever been the listener who did not pay close attention. Tell students that listening for critical information at home or in the community is important just like it is at school.

LESSON ACTIVITIES

1. Have students sit or stand in a circle. Tell students that they will practice listening for critical information about each other. Each student should think of something he or she is an expert at. Each student will need to tell two things that helped him or her become an expert. Start the game by relating your expertise (e.g., you are an expert at growing orchids), two things that helped you become an expert, and then pass the ball to a student. This first student will need to tell what your skill is and how you became good at it, and then tell about his or her own special skill and how he or she became good at it. The student will then toss the ball to someone else in the circle, who repeats only the previous student's skill followed by his or her own. Students should listen carefully since they will never know when they might have to relate the critical information they have heard. If necessary, allow students to write critical information down as this is clearly a strategy for dealing with critical information. Keep passing the ball until everyone has had a turn.

2. After the activity is finished, let students discuss how it made them feel to have others listen and tell something special about them. Have students relate their feelings to family members and friends. Effective listeners help others feel good about themselves.

3. Brainstorm ideas about signals for identifying critical information at home and in the community. Have students consider signals from friends and family members. Write ideas where everyone can see them. Summarize by referring to the *Identifying Signals* poster. When critical information is missed, the consequences can effect your friendships or your relationships with family members. Point out that one strategy for dealing with critical information is to "Take action! Write it down!"

4. Hand out *Rapid Write: Critical Information (Part II)*. Read through the directions as a group and check for understanding. Give students time to write two examples of critical information they might receive at home and two possible consequences for missing critical information. Repeat this process for critical information in a community setting. Discuss their different responses.

CLOSURE

Summarize the lesson, review its relevance to students, and tie it to future learning. Have students name a few signals that let them know a friend is about to tell something critical. Remind them that identifying the signal can help them remember to "Take Action! Write It Down!" Review examples of critical information at home and in the community. Tell students that in the next lesson *(Static: Listening for Relevance [Part I])* the idea of critical information will be taken to another level; they will have to use critical information to make decisions about whether what they hear or read is relevant to them.

Rapid Write

CRITICAL INFORMATION (PART II)

Date: ____________________________

Name: ____

Directions

- My job is to write 2 examples of when I might listen for critical information at home and in the community. Then I'll write possible consequences for not identifying critical information in each situation.
- I'll need this paper and a pencil.
- I'll know I'm finished when I have written 8 complete sentences.
- When I'm finished I'll share this work with the teacher.

Write examples of when you might hear critical information and consequences for missing that information.

I might hear critical information at home when:

1. ____
2. ____

If I miss critical information at home with family members, these are possible consequences:

1. ____
2. ____

I might hear critical information in the community when:

1. ____
2. ____

If I miss critical information in the community, these are possible consequences:

1. ____
2. ____

© 2001 *Thinking Publications.* Duplication permitted for educational use only.

STATIC: LISTENING FOR RELEVANCE (PART I)

GOAL

To tune in relevant information and tune out irrelevant information

BACKGROUND INFORMATION

The purpose of this lesson is to introduce the terms *relevant* and *irrelevant.* The lesson encourages students to listen for critical information and then determine if it is relevant to them. Students draw conclusions or make inferences from the presented material to help decide if the information is related to the current topic and is relevant to them. A differentiation between critical (i.e., important facts to remember) and relevant (i.e., appropriate for or related to the situation) should be made for students. Irrelevant information is introduced as one or more forms of "static" that can interfere with students' ability to stay tuned in to the important signal (i.e., the speaker or the topic).

Static: Listening for Relevance (Part II) provides an opportunity to listen actively and determine sound effects to be added to a play script. In *Static: Listening for Relevance (Part III),* students listen for extended periods of time with the addition of distractors in a radio show production.

OBJECTIVES

1. Understand the terms *relevant* and *irrelevant.*
2. Listen for relevant information.
3. Distinguish relevant from irrelevant information.

MATERIALS

1. *Tune Out the Irrelevant! Tune In the Relevant!* graphic (See page 37; duplicate and enlarge the graphic, color it, mount it onto construction paper or poster board, and laminate it for durability if desired.)
2. *Rapid Write: Static (Part I)* (See page 38; duplicate one per student.)

INTRODUCTION

Tie-in to Prior Learning

Remind students that in the previous lesson (*Critical Information: Identifying Signals [Part II]*) they identified signals for critical information in oral or written form. Ask students to give examples of critical and noncritical information. Explain that in this lesson they will have the opportunity to practice this skill in a different way by discussing how critical information can become unimportant depending on the situation.

Focus/Relevance

Ask students if they have ever had trouble tuning in to a clear signal on the radio. When they listened to a poorly tuned station, the static on the radio could have been caused by several different signals coming in at one time or by being too far away from the source to get one clear signal. Discuss the different kinds of static that can occur in a classroom that could interfere with learning: object static (e.g., playing with materials), people static (e.g., neighbors talking), body static (e.g., hunger or physical needs), or even idea static (e.g., thinking about other things). Tell students that anything that interferes with learning could be considered static and needs to be tuned out or ignored. Explain that in this lesson they will be discovering that a situation sometimes helps determine whether information is static (i.e., irrelevant) or if it is relevant.

LESSON ACTIVITIES

1. Read the following examples of possible announcements students might hear over the intercom. Have students signal by raising their hands if they think the message would be important for them to tune in to.

    - The lunch menu for today includes pizza, salad, green beans, and fruit.
    - Teachers have a faculty meeting after school that they must attend.
    - All students must attend the pep rally at 1:00 this afternoon.

    Discuss their responses. Explain that some examples contained critical information but were unimportant to them (i.e., irrelevant) and some contained critical information that was important to them (i.e., relevant). Use these examples to explain the difference between critical and relevant. Discuss other examples generated by students to ensure comprehension of vocabulary.

2. Show the *Tune Out the Irrelevant! Tune In the Relevant!* poster. Tell students that static is a kind of interference. Refer back to the focus section and the radio signals, highlighting each type of static on the poster. To block out static, tell students that they must keep their brains tuned in to the important, relevant signal. Remind students that when someone makes a comment that is not about the discussion topic, they are creating static or interference by bringing up an irrelevant topic. Give this example of a class discussing the planets in the solar system:

    > *Lots of students are raising their hands to comment, ask questions, or to add information and one student raises a hand and says, "Next Monday my grandparents are coming for a visit."*

The irrelevant comment brought the discussion to a halt. Emphasize that it is important to stay relevant in a discussion, and to not share irrelevant information or contribute static. Practice determining relevance with the following announcements by having students signal with a thumbs-up response if they think the information is relevant to them and a thumbs-down if it is irrelevant. Ask them to defend each response.

- Today, information on the school carnival will be sent home to parents with the oldest child.
- If you are going to middle school next year (or substitute an appropriate grade level), there will be an orientation for your parents on Thursday evening.
- If you submitted a history project, please report to the library after school.
- Kindergartners and first graders will be attending a puppet show at 10:00 a.m.
- Please be sure to lock up your bicycles.
- Those who have turned in their daily work may have computer time or an activity of their choice.
- Because today is an "ozone alert" day there is no outdoor sports practice.

Summarize this activity by pointing out that the situation can determine if the information is relevant to you.

3. Tell students that they are going to have an opportunity to practice listening for relevant versus irrelevant information. Divide students into two teams. One team will speak first while the other team listens and evaluates the comments for relevance. Choose a topic for conversation, such as one of the following:

   - What is your favorite type of dog and why?
   - What is your favorite subject in school and why?
   - What is the best book you have ever read and why?
   - Do you like vanilla or chocolate ice cream the best and why?
   - What is your favorite sport and why?
   - If you could create a new extracurricular activity at school, what would it be and why?

   Each person on the speaking team makes a comment about the topic. When the team makes five relevant comments in a row, they gain a point. Meanwhile, the listening team should be evaluating whether or not the comments are relevant. If they catch an irrelevant comment, and can defend their opinion, they gain a point for their team.

4. Point out that relevance is important in both spoken and written language. Create a graphic organizer and place it where everyone can see it. For example, use a graphic web to represent

one of the topics discussed. Write the topic in a center circle with rays drawn outward from the center to represent each relevant comment. A graphic organizer is useful for stressing that supporting details pertain to the topic and relevant comments can be combined in writing assignments to form paragraphs.

5. Hand out *Rapid Write: Static (Part I)*. Read through the directions as a group and check for understanding. Give students time to write two sentences that are relevant to each topic given. Discuss their responses.

CLOSURE

Summarize the lesson, review its relevance to students, and tie it to future learning. Remind students that relevance is determined by the situation. Tell students that in the next lesson *(Static: Listening for Relevance [Part II])* they will be listening for relevant details from a story. They will be determining sound effects that might be relevant to the story to help listeners picture the story events in their mind as they listen to a radio show performance.

Tune Out the Irrelevant! Tune In the Relevant!

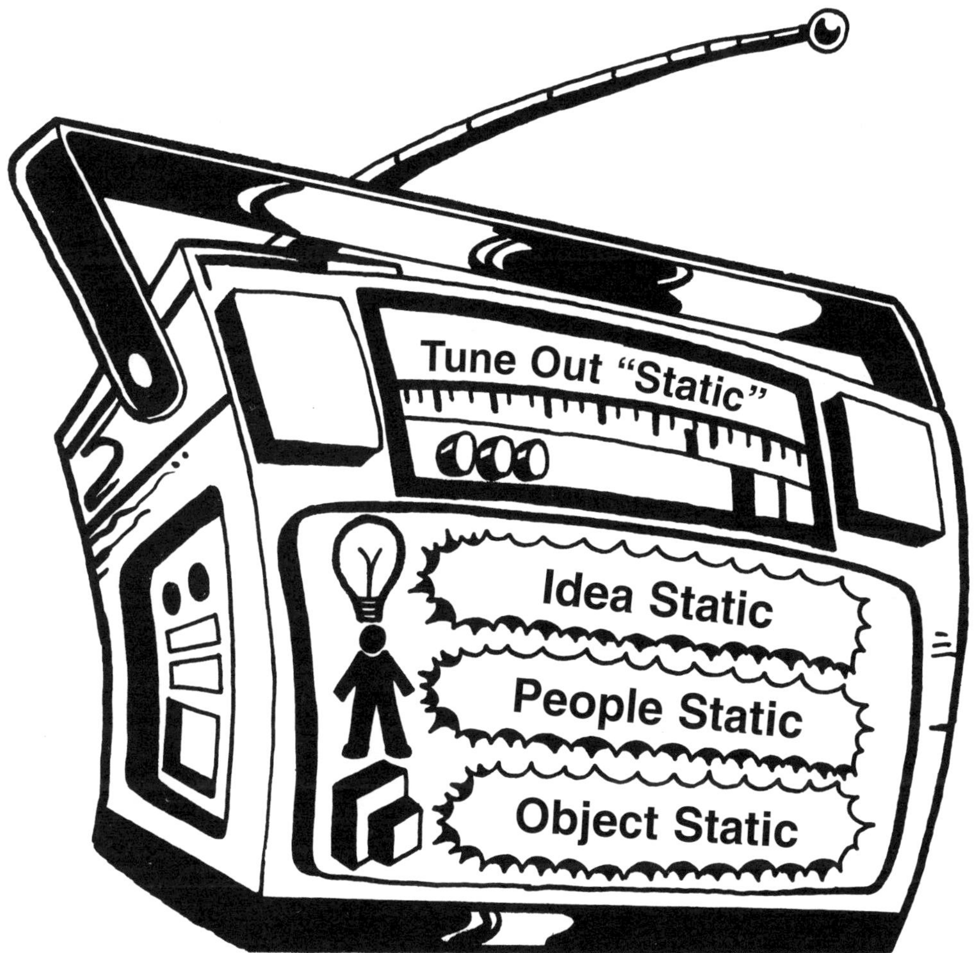

Relevant information is:

Related to your family, friends, and school	Related to the topic	Changes with the situation

© 2001 *Thinking Publications.* Duplication permitted for educational use only.

RAPID WRITE

STATIC (PART I)

Date: ______________________

Name: ______________________________

Directions

- My job is to write 2 sentences that are relevant to each topic.
- I'll need this paper and a pencil.
- I'll know I'm finished when I have written 4 complete sentences with correct punctuation.
- When I'm finished I'll share this work with the teacher.

Write two ideas that are relevant to each topic.

- Football is an exciting sport.

1. ______________________________

____

2. ______________________________

____

- Pets are a big responsibility.

1. ______________________________

____

2. ______________________________

____

© 2001 *Thinking Publications.* Duplication permitted for educational use only.

STATIC: LISTENING FOR RELEVANCE (PART II)

GOAL

To tune in relevant information and tune out irrelevant information

BACKGROUND INFORMATION

In *Static: Listening for Relevance (Part I),* students learned the terms *relevant* and *irrelevant* and practiced identifying relevant statements about a given topic. The purpose of this lesson is to have students listen carefully to a story and think of sound effects that might be relevant in a play script based on the story. Students will listen to a story to prepare for the production of a radio show. They will evaluate and decide on sound effects that might be relevant for listeners to understand and enjoy the radio show. In *Static: Listening for Relevance (Part III),* students will have an opportunity to listen actively for extended periods of time with the addition of distractors presented in a radio show production.

OBJECTIVES

1. Understand the importance of identifying relevant information.
2. Listen for relevant information.
3. Use information from a story to make inferences, draw conclusions, and determine relevance.
4. Maintain relevance to a topic while discussing ideas within a group.

MATERIALS

1. *Bubba the Cowboy Prince: A Fractured Texas Tale* (1997) by Helen Ketteman (This book was selected because of the variety of interesting characters, use of figurative language, simple story line, and opportunities for sound effects. Any book with similar characteristics can be substituted.)
2. *Tune Out the Irrelevant! Tune In the Relevant!* poster (Created earlier)
3. *Rapid Write: Static (Part II)* (See page 42; duplicate one per student.)

INTRODUCTION

Tie-in to Prior Learning

Remind students that in the last lesson *(Static: Listening for Relevance [Part I])* they discussed the terms *relevant* and *irrelevant* and discovered that relevance can change with the situation. Tell students that it is important to avoid bringing up irrelevant information and to tune out information that creates static and keeps them from learning.

Focus/Relevance

Ask students to raise their hand if they have ever read a script or performed in a play. Share ideas about what is involved in putting on a performance (e.g., rehearsing, listening for cues, and inflecting your voice). Tell students that they will be producing a radio show in this lesson (*Part II*) and the next lesson (*Part III*). The objective in this lesson will be to stay tuned in to the story and identify possible sound effects for their radio show performance.

LESSON ACTIVITIES

1. Highlight the difference between listening and hearing. Tell students that during the school day, they are continuously exposed to information, either spoken or written. It would be impossible to remember everything they hear or read in a day, so they have to identify information that is relevant. Explain to students that identifying relevant information may help them do better at school, make wiser decisions, keep safe, get rewards, make friends, and keep friends.

2. Tell students that you are going to read a book to them and they will be making a radio show based on the story you read. Discuss how a radio performance might be different from a TV show, movie, or play. Explain that the first part of the production activity will be to listen to the story that the script will be based on and identify situations in the story that could be produced with sound effects. Cue students to think of sound effects that enhance the listener's understanding of the story and are relevant to the story. Stress that they can help their listeners picture the scene and actions by the way they speak their lines and by choosing relevant sound effects.

3. Before reading *Bubba the Cowboy Prince: A Fractured Texas Tale,* show the cover of the book and discuss the author and illustrator. Tell students that this story is adapted from a very familiar fairy tale. Ask if they can identify the fairy tale just by looking at the cover. Ask students to predict what the author might mean by subtitling the story *A Fractured Texas Tale.* As you read the story, tell students to listen for where sound effects might go best so that a list can be generated after the story is read.

4. Read the story. Highlight the following literary components:

   - Setting—discuss and note how the dialect, illustrations, and writing styles depict a rural setting
   - Vocabulary—*strapping, doggies, cow patties, purtiest, spread, duds, bolo tie, fetch, cud, hoedown, Stetson, dude, lumbered, ruckus, aim, obliged*

- Figurative language—*cute as a cow's ear, throw a ball, gussied up, sorrier than a steer in a stockyard, lower than a rattlesnake in a gully, darker than a black bull at midnight, a Texas thunderstorm was brewing, bonked the bejeebers out of his bean, whiter than a new salt lick, mite familiar, winning her heart, looked sorry, chicken fits*

5. After reading the story, brainstorm possible sound effects that might be relevant to the story. Examples include running feet, a polishing sound, water splashing, a climbing into a wagon sound, sighs, cows mooing, a rattlesnake tail rattling, wind, thunder, chewing, sucking, smacking, a magical sound, horse neighs, hooves stomping, a clock ticking, sniffing, yawning, and music.

6. Refer students to the *Tune Out the Irrelevant! Tune In the Relevant!* poster, and remind them that they will practice this strategy in the next lesson *(Static: Listening for Relevance [Part III])* as they determine instruments to make sound effects, rehearse their parts, and record the radio show.

7. Hand out *Rapid Write: Static (Part II)*. Read through the directions as a group and check for understanding. Ask students to list 10 possible sound effects that would be relevant to the story. Discuss their responses. As a group, decide which sound effects you will use. Write them where everyone can see them, and save them for use in *Static: Listening for Relevance (Part III)*. Encourage students to tune out the irrelevant and tune in the relevant information as you have this discussion.

CLOSURE

Summarize the lesson, review its relevance to students, and tie it to future learning. Remind students that they have developed a list of sound effects for the play script in the next lesson *(Static: Listening for Relevance [Part III])*. Ask them to think more about how they will make each sound (e.g., using certain instruments).

RAPID WRITE

STATIC (PART II)

Date: ______________________

Name: ______________________________________

Directions

- My job is to list sound effects that might be used during events in the play script.
- I'll need this paper and a pencil.
- I'll know I'm finished when I have written 10 sound effects.
- When I'm finished I'll share this work with the teacher.

Make a list of possible sound effects for the story.

1. ______________________________
2. ______________________________
3. ______________________________
4. ______________________________
5. ______________________________
6. ______________________________
7. ______________________________
8. ______________________________
9. ______________________________
10. ______________________________

© 2001 *Thinking Publications.* Duplication permitted for educational use only.

STATIC: LISTENING FOR RELEVANCE (PART III)

GOAL

To tune in relevant information and tune out irrelevant information

BACKGROUND INFORMATION

In *Part I* and *Part II* of *Static: Listening for Relevance,* students learned about relevant and irrelevant information. The purpose of this lesson is to provide students with an opportunity to listen for extended periods of time with the addition of distractors. The distractors in this lesson are both physical (props) and environmental (neighbors with props, a variety of speakers, scripts, and sound effects).

Students will produce a radio show based on the story *Bubba the Cowboy Prince: A Fractured Texas Tale.* Before producing the radio show, students will evaluate and decide how the various sound effects can be made. Students will listen to ideas, discuss the pros and cons of each idea objectively and politely, and select the ideas that will have the most relevance to the show. They can also defend their choices for sound effects by writing or sharing supporting reasons for their choice.

OBJECTIVES

1. Listen for relevant information.
2. Tune in to auditory cues to read lines from the script or perform actions.
3. Maintain relevance to a topic while discussing ideas within a group.

MATERIALS

1. *Bubba Script* (See pages 46–51; duplicate one per student and prepare one overhead transparency. The script provided is an adaptation of the dialogue from this book. If you used a different story in *Static: Listening for Relevance (Part II),* you will need to create a similar script. Also note that the example sound effect instruments listed relate to *Bubba the Cowboy Prince.*)
2. List of sound effects (Created in *Part II*)
3. *Rapid Write: Static (Part III)* (See page 52; duplicate one per student and prepare one overhead transparency.)
4. Sound effects objects and instruments (e.g., xylophone, gong, and sandpaper blocks)
5. *Tune Out the Irrelevant! Tune In the Relevant!* poster (Created earlier)

INTRODUCTION

Tie-in to Prior Learning

Remind students that in the last lesson *(Static: Listening for Relevance [Part II])* they listened to the story *Bubba the Cowboy Prince* and brainstormed relevant sound effects to use in a radio show production.

Focus/Relevance

Tell students they have an important job in this lesson because they will be both directors and actors for the radio show. Remind them that the director has a very important role to play because he or she must set the stage for the entire production and pay close attention to whether the sound effects are relevant. Remind the actors that they are responsible for making the sound effects at appropriate times.

LESSON ACTIVITIES

1. Hand out the *Bubba Script* and assign parts. Students without a part can be in charge of sound effects. Read through the script as a group, and stop when students feel a sound effect could be used. Refer to the list of sound effects created in *Part II*. Have each student write the sound effect in the "Sound Effect" column on their scripts. Writing on an overhead transparency of the *Bubba Script* will help students follow along.

2. Display the overhead of *Rapid Write: Static (Part III)*. Read through the directions as a group and check for understanding. Assign different sound effects to different students. Have students write ideas for creating their assigned sound effects on their *Rapid Write* page. Tell students to use complete sentences to describe how the sound will be made and to explain its relevance to the performance. The writing could be done individually or in small groups.

   HINT: Remind students that the music teacher may have instruments that could be borrowed for the radio show.

3. Return to the *Bubba Script* and decide who will make each sound effect or when the entire group will make a sound effect. Have students gather or make their sound effects and practice using them. During this working session, remind students to tune out irrelevant information and tune in relevant information to complete their work in a timely way. Refer to the *Tune Out the Irrelevant! Tune In the Relevant!* poster for this purpose.

4. Have characters read their parts while sound effects are practiced. Model or role-play giving and receiving compliments or suggestions as different students read their character's part (e.g., "I like the way Susan is using a special voice to sound like Miz Lurleen"). Demonstrate the

phrase "Why don't you try..." as another way to offer suggestions in a positive way. Praise or reinforce members of the group as they give and receive compliments or suggestions and as they tune in to relevant information. Help sound effect "technicians" learn cues that signal their part.

5. Record the performance of the radio show.
6. Listen to the performance and evaluate it with students. Allow them to share compliments with each other on their respective performances.

CLOSURE

Summarize the lesson, review its relevance to students, and tie it to future learning. Compliment students on their hard work, their improvement in listening, and their appropriate use of suggestions and compliments that resulted in a wonderful performance. Remind them that they learned a lot in the last few lessons about relevance and its importance in daily communication. Tell students that in the next lesson *(Hit the Bull's-Eye: Evaluating Directions [Part I])* they will be practicing a skill that they use every day.

BUBBA SCRIPT

Characters:

- Narrator
- Miz Lurleen
- Dwayne
- Stepdaddy
- Milton
- Fairy godcow
- Bubba

		Sound Effect
Narrator:	Once upon a time, way out West, there lived a wiry young cowpoke named Bubba. He lived on a ranch with his ornery stepdaddy and his hateful and lazy stepbrothers, Dwayne and Milton.	
Bubba:	I work from dawn to dusk doing the chores of three ranch hands but I'm not complaining. I love ranching!	
Narrator:	Dwayne and Milton would sit on their horses and boss poor Bubba around.	
Dwayne:	Hey, Bubba, move them doggies along there. Time's a wastin'!	
Milton:	Yeah, and watch out for cow patties! You know Daddy hates fer you to track up the house.	
Narrator:	Now, down the road a piece lived Miz Lurleen. She was finer than frog hair—and that's mighty fine—and rich to boot! She owned the biggest spread south of the Red River.	
Miz Lurleen:	I just love the ranching life, but it can be a might lonely. I think it's time to find myself a cowpoke who will love ranching as much as I do. And it wouldn't hurt if he was cute as a bug either. I'm going to throw a hoedown bigger than a Texas twister and invite all the ranchers.	

© 2001 *Thinking Publications.* Duplication permitted for educational use only.

Narrator: And she did. Soon the day of the shindig arrived. Milton and Dwayne spent all day bossing Bubba around. He had to help them get all gussied up in their finest duds. Bubba just about ran himself ragged waiting on the two of them.

Dwayne: Bubba, fetch my Stetson hat!

Milton: Bubba, git my boots polished pronto!

Stepdaddy: Bubba, brush them horses and wash that wagon!

Narrator: After waiting on Dwayne and Milton and Stepdaddy, Bubba was exhausted. But still he asked, as they climbed into the wagon...

Bubba: Can't you wait for me to get ready? I want to do some boot-scootin' with Miz Lurleen too.

Dwayne, Milton, Stepdaddy: *[hoot and holler]*

Milton: Miz Lurleen wouldn't dance with the likes of you! Why, your shirt's too raggedy and dirty to even clean her boots.

Dwayne: You're sorrier than a steer in a stockyard.

Stepdaddy: The cattle wouldn't even want to stand too close to you! They would smell you from across the pasture and run!

Narrator: Bubba looked into the mirror and saw that it was true.

Bubba: I don't have a respectable shirt to wear. My boots are downright disgraceful. I guess I could do with a dunk in the tub and some purty perfumed soap! Milton and Dwayne are right. Miz Lurleen wouldn't dance with the likes of me.

© 2001 *Thinking Publications*. Duplication permitted for educational use only.

Sound Effect

Narrator: Bubba hung his head. He felt lower than a rattlesnake in a rabbit hole. As Milton, Dwayne, and Stepdaddy went on off to the ball, Bubba headed for the pasture to check on the herd. Meanwhile, dark clouds began to gather on the horizon. It looked like a Texas thunderstorm was brewing. Suddenly, as Bubba approached the pasture, a bolt of lightning struck and knocked him to the ground. For a moment, Bubba was dazed and confused, but then he heard a voice.

Fairy godcow: Go to the ball, Bubba.

Narrator: Bubba looked around. There was no one there except him and the cows.

Bubba: I must have knocked the stuffin' out of my head 'cause I'd swear that cow just talked to me.

Narrator: The cow chewed her cud for a moment.

Fairy godcow: I'm your fairy godcow and I'm here to help you go to the hoedown.

Narrator: Bubba sat up rubbing his head.

Bubba: I was aimin' to go, but shucks, I don't have a thing to wear.

Narrator: The fairy godcow swished her tail, and Bubba's raggedy clothes changed into the finest cowboy duds he'd ever seen. He looked down to see starched blue jeans, shiny new black boots, and a sparkling white shirt with a Stetson hat to match.

© 2001 *Thinking Publications.* Duplication permitted for educational use only.

Bubba: Why I look downright purty!

Narrator: The fairy godcow swished her tail again, and a nearby steer turned into the most beautiful white charger Bubba had ever seen.

Fairy godcow: Now, you go on to the dance, Bubba, and have a good time dancing with Miz Lurleen. But you'd better get back home before midnight 'cause that's when the magic runs out.

Bubba: Yahoo!

Narrator: Bubba jumped on his horse and raced off to the party. When Bubba arrived, the ballroom was hoppin'. But every time Miz Lurleen finished a dance, she just yawned.

Miz Lurleen: These fellas couldn't fill the boots of a real cowboy if they were all wearin' the same pair!

Narrator: By the time it was Bubba's turn to dance with Miz Lurleen, it was almost midnight. Soon as she saw Bubba, Miz Lurleen's eyes lit up.

Miz Lurleen: Why you're cuter than a newborn calf!

Narrator: Bubba blushed and then took Miz Lurleen in his arms and started sashaying across the dance floor. Dwayne and Milton were so jealous they turned several shades of green.

Dwayne: Who is that dude?

Milton: I don't recall seeing him around these parts before, but there is something about him that looks a mite familiar.

© 2001 *Thinking Publications.* Duplication permitted for educational use only.

Sound Effect

Stepdaddy: Don't just stand there! That cowboy's about to capture Miz Lurleen's affections.

Narrator: As it turned out, Milton and Dwayne didn't have to do a thing, because right in the middle of Bubba and Miz Lurleen's do-si-do, the clock struck midnight. Suddenly Bubba's fancy outfit turned into the dirty rags he usually wore around the ranch. He looked pitiful and he smelled even worse.

Milton: What is that dreadful odor?

Dwayne: Why, it's Bubba!

Bubba: I'm, I'm, m-m-mighty sorry, Miz Lurleen!

Narrator: Bubba turned bright red and raced out of the room.

Miz Lurleen: Don't go!

Narrator: But Bubba didn't waste any time. He leaped on his cow and lumbered off into the night. Bubba lost one of his dirty cowboy boots during all the commotion. Miz Lurleen grabbed the boot and stood clutching it in her arms.

Miz Lurleen: This is the boot of a real cowboy, and I aim to marry the man who can fill this shoe!

Narrator: Miz Lurleen went back inside and began to ask everybody at the ball who the mysterious cowboy was. Nobody had a clue except Dwayne, Milton, and Stepdaddy but they weren't talking. Starting early the next morning, Miz Lurleen

© 2001 *Thinking Publications.* Duplication permitted for educational use only.

went from ranch to ranch, searching for the cowboy who could fill that boot. When she came to Dwayne and Milton's ranch, both brothers tried the boot on, but they just couldn't squeeze into it. Miz Lurleen was just about to leave when Bubba rode up. He looked like he had been wrestling with pigs in a wallow and he smelled even worse. To top it all off, he was only wearing one boot. Miz Lurleen jumped off her horse and ran over to Bubba and hollered...

Miz Lurleen: Try this on!

Narrator: Bubba took the dirty old boot and pulled it on. It fit like a glove.

Bubba: I'm mighty grateful, ma'am.

Miz Lurleen: You're the cowpoke of my dreams! I'd know that smell anywhere! Marry me, big fella, and help me work my ranch.

Narrator: Meanwhile, Dwayne, Milton, and Stepdaddy were having a fit. But Bubba just grinned as he and Miz Lurleen rode off into the sunset. They lived happily ever after, roping, cowpoking, and getting them doggies along!

© 2001 *Thinking Publications.* Duplication permitted for educational use only.

RAPID WRITE

STATIC (PART III)

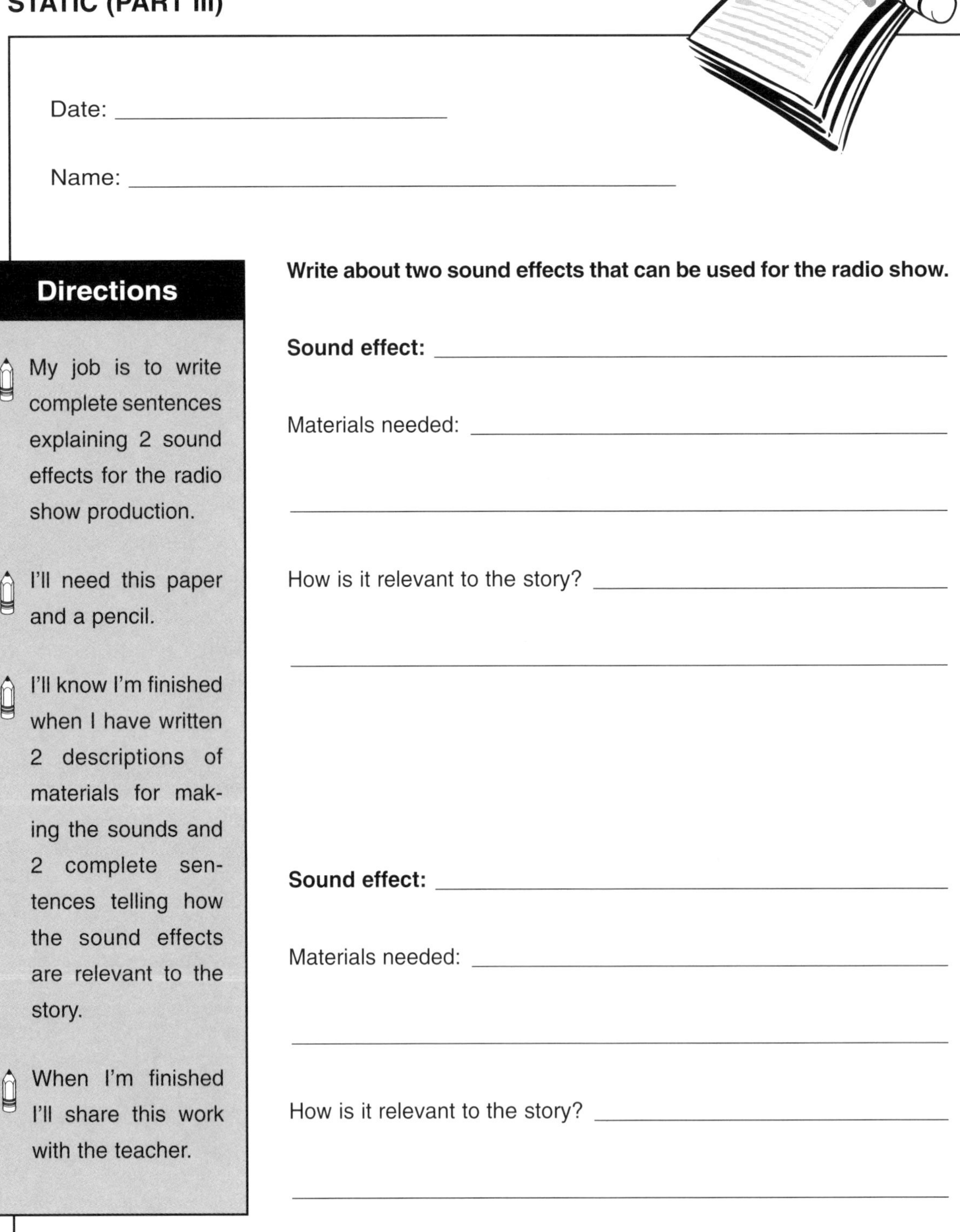

Date: ____________________

Name: ______________________________

Directions

- My job is to write complete sentences explaining 2 sound effects for the radio show production.
- I'll need this paper and a pencil.
- I'll know I'm finished when I have written 2 descriptions of materials for making the sounds and 2 complete sentences telling how the sound effects are relevant to the story.
- When I'm finished I'll share this work with the teacher.

Write about two sound effects that can be used for the radio show.

Sound effect: ______________________________

Materials needed: ______________________________

____

How is it relevant to the story? ______________________________

____

Sound effect: ______________________________

Materials needed: ______________________________

____

How is it relevant to the story? ______________________________

____

© 2001 *Thinking Publications.* Duplication permitted for educational use only.

HIT THE BULL'S-EYE: EVALUATING DIRECTIONS (PART I)

GOAL

To give and receive directions

BACKGROUND INFORMATION

The purpose of this lesson is to evaluate given information, whether spoken or written. It encourages students to ask the questions "Does it make sense? Do I need more information? Is it a reasonable request?" When evaluating directions, students must first learn how to give and receive specific, detailed directions so that they know how to repair a communication breakdown.

Part I requires the use of barrier game boards and game pieces. A barrier game has some type of obstruction or shield between the speaker and the listener so each cannot see what the other is doing. After one or more directions are given, either orally or in writing, the barrier is removed and the listener and speaker analyze whether a communication breakdown occurred. In the next lesson (*Part II*), students will continue to practice evaluating directions while drawing conclusions about the information given and apply this strategy to life skills.

OBJECTIVES

1. Understand the terms *clarification* and *reference points.*
2. Ask for clarification when given insufficient directions or information.
3. Give clear and precise directions using specific vocabulary.

MATERIALS

1. Barrier game packets (Create one packet per student. Create the game board by duplicating the landscape on pages 57–58, gluing it onto a file folder, coloring it and laminating the file folder for durability. Duplicate *Barrier Game Pieces* from pages 59–60, color them, laminate them, cut them out, and place them in an envelope or plastic bag for each student.)
2. *Evaluate Directions to Hit the Bull's-Eye!* graphic (See page 56; duplicate and enlarge the graphic, color it, mount it onto construction paper or poster board, and laminate it for durability if desired.)
3. *Direction Strips* (See pages 61–62; duplicate one set per student, copy the strips onto heavy stock paper, cut them apart, laminate for durability if desired, and place them in envelopes.)

4. Objects to act as barriers (e.g., books, binders, and boxes)
5. *Rapid Write: Hit the Bull's-Eye (Part I)* (See page 63; duplicate one per student.)

INTRODUCTION

Tie-in to Prior Learning

Review how to listen effectively from the previous lessons *(Parts I, II,* and *III* of *Static: Listening for Relevance)* when students had to tune in to relevant information and tune out the irrelevant "static" to prepare for and perform a radio show. Explain that students are now ready to send and receive their own clear signals.

Focus/Relevance

1. Tell students that you are about to put a lot of "object static" on their desks and you want them to tune it out and listen to your critical signal. Give each student a barrier game packet (i.e., a game board and a bag of game pieces).
2. Tell students that you will be giving them some directions to follow using the game board and pieces. Remind them not to ask any questions but follow the directions as best they can. Purposely give imprecise directions (e.g., "Put the tree in the grass" or "Put the volcano on the side"). Lead students to discover that imprecise directions can break down communication by comparing their inconsistent placements of game pieces on the game boards.

Lesson Activities

1. Ask students if they had difficulty following the directions and why. Show the *Evaluate Directions to Hit the Bull's-Eye!* poster and discuss the need for clarification when directions do not make sense, when directions do not give enough information, or when a request is unreasonable. Define the word *clarification.* Elicit the idea that clarifying directions makes information exactly right, just like when an arrow hits the center of a target (i.e., the bull's-eye). Highlight the strategies for "Listening/Reading" and "Speaking/Writing" on the poster. Discuss the need for understanding the vocabulary in directions and using precise direction words. Explain how to use reference points, like objects or landmarks, when giving directions. Explain that when a communication breakdown occurs, students could follow one or all of the following steps:
   - Ask for clarification and specific vocabulary—"Excuse me, did you mean the pine tree, the pear tree, or the apple tree?" Stress that students need to use specific vocabulary when giving directions and that if they do not understand a word when hearing directions, they should ask for clarification.

- Reread for clarity—Identify the "chunks" of information in the directions, and tell students that when information is chunked together in pieces it breaks the directions down into easier steps to remember and follow.
- Ask for more precise direction words and reference points—Remind them to use a *reference point,* an object or a landmark that will give further information in the directions (e.g., "Put the lake in the southeast corner near the waterfall"). Point out the compass. Discuss the use of direction words such as north, south, east, west, to the right of, to the left of, above, below, and on top.
- Jot it down—Tell students that when directions get confusing or too long to remember, writing keywords down can help (e.g., "Just a minute, please. Let me write some keywords down").

2. Before playing the barrier games, hand out *Direction Strips* to each student and have students take turns reading them. The readers must decide if the information on the strip makes sense, provides enough information, and provides specific directions that can be followed. For some directions, students may need to reread the strip several times to find the chunks of information that can be given as separate steps. Give assistance as needed by helping readers clarify directions that need to be more specific—making the directions exactly right, like hitting the bull's-eye.
3. To play the barrier games, have students work in pairs, using a book or some other object as a barrier between them and their game boards. Students should alternate being the speaker and the listener. Tell students to take turns giving three specific directions to their partner. Point out that the first thing they might do is place their compass on the game board (with N pointing to the top of the landscape). When one partner has given three directions, tell students to remove the barrier and compare the pieces on their game boards. When all students have played both roles, discuss how they did. Remind them to use the strategies from the *Evaluate Directions to Hit the Bull's-Eye!* poster (i.e., ask for clarification, use specific vocabulary, reread for clarity, use direction words, jot it down, and give reference points) when giving and receiving directions to each other.
4. Hand out *Rapid Write: Hit the Bull's-Eye (Part I)*. Read through the directions as a group and check for understanding. Have students write three new directions for placing objects on the landscape folder. Remind students to reread for clarity before asking for help or finishing their work. Let students share their directions with the class as time allows. Discuss the need for clarification.

CLOSURE

Summarize the lesson, review its relevance to students, and tie it to future learning. Ask students why they are able to "hit the bull's-eye" now but were not as successful at the beginning of the lesson. Elicit the idea that they can now evaluate directions, ask for clarification, use specific vocabulary, reread for clarity, use direction words, give reference points, and jot down keywords when giving or receiving directions.

Evaluate Directions to Hit the Bull's-Eye!

DOES IT MAKE SENSE?
DO I NEED MORE INFORMATION?
IS IT A REASONABLE REQUEST?
EVALUATING...
BULL'S-EYE!

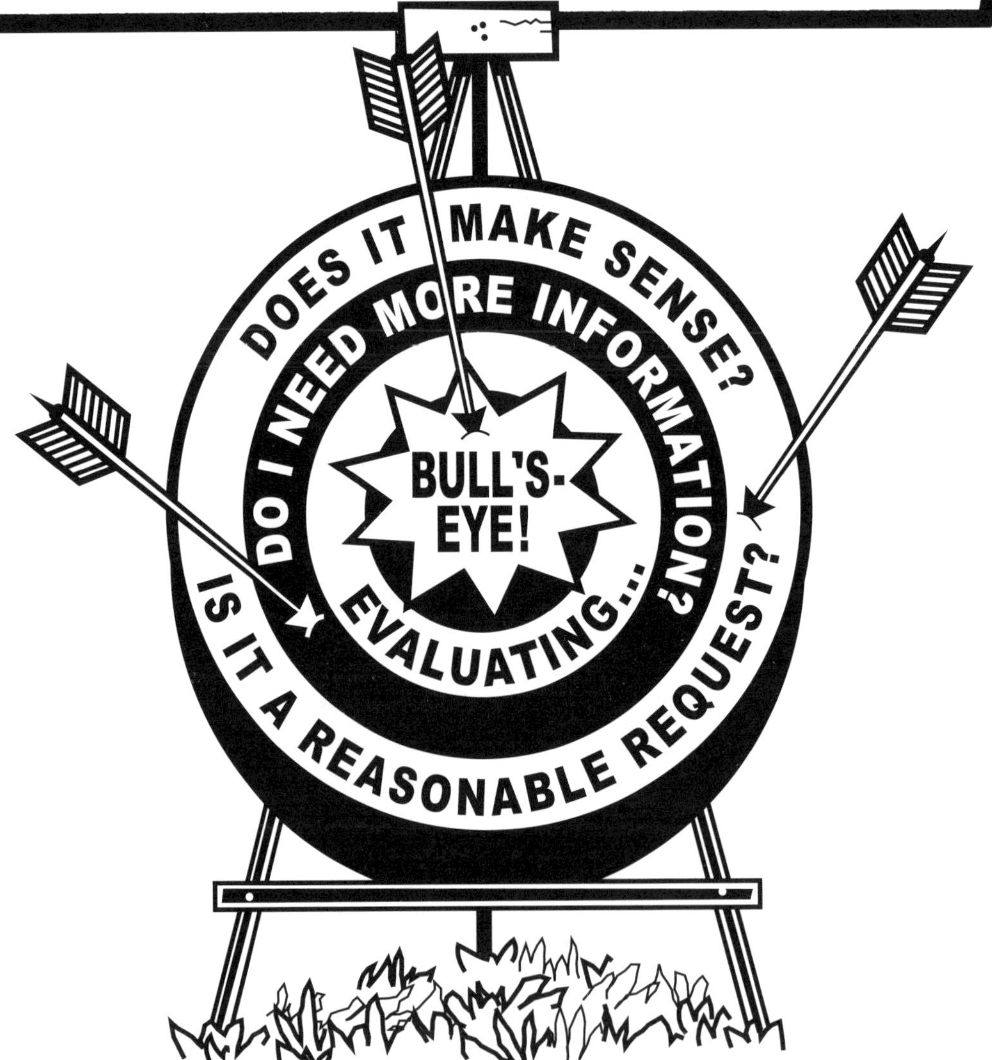

Listening/Reading	Speaking/Writing
Request clarification	Use specific vocabulary
Reread for clarity	Use direction words
Jot it down	Give reference points

© 2001 *Thinking Publications.* Duplication permitted for educational use only.

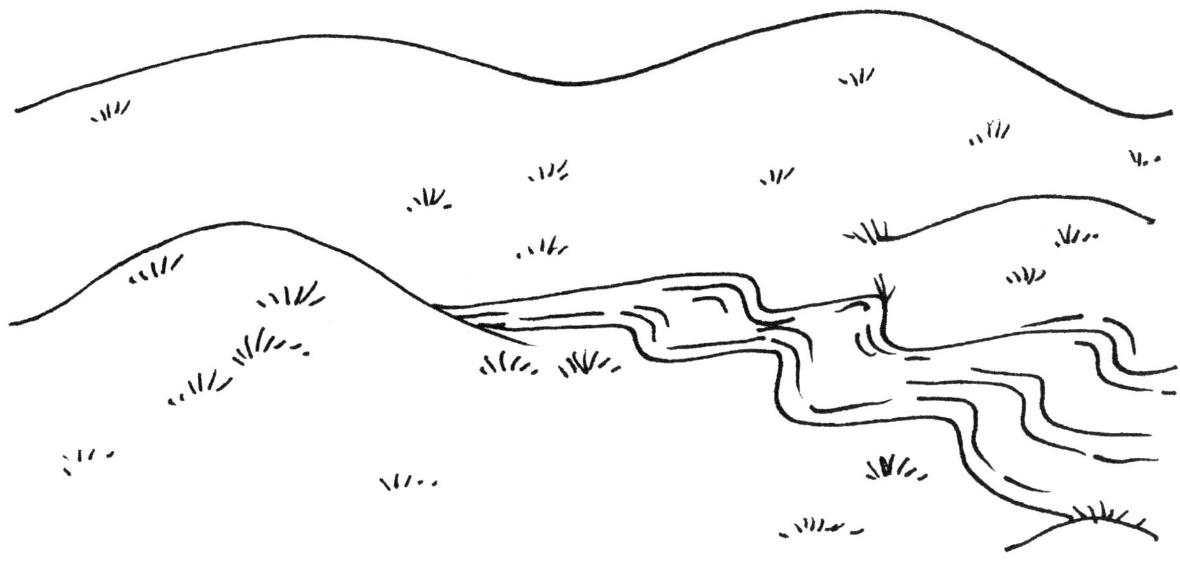

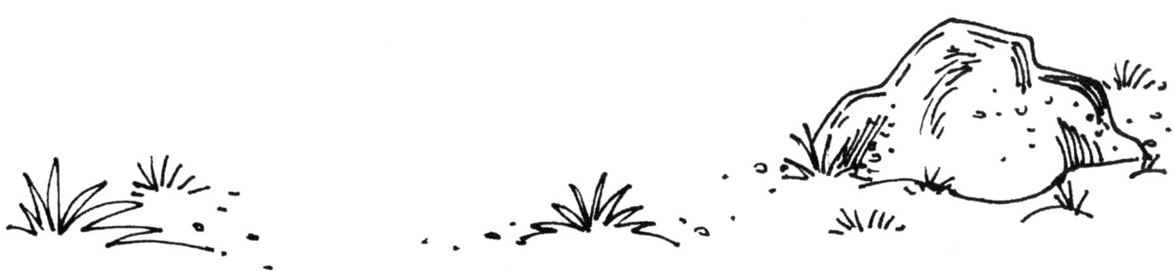

© 2001 *Thinking Publications.* Duplication permitted for educational use only.

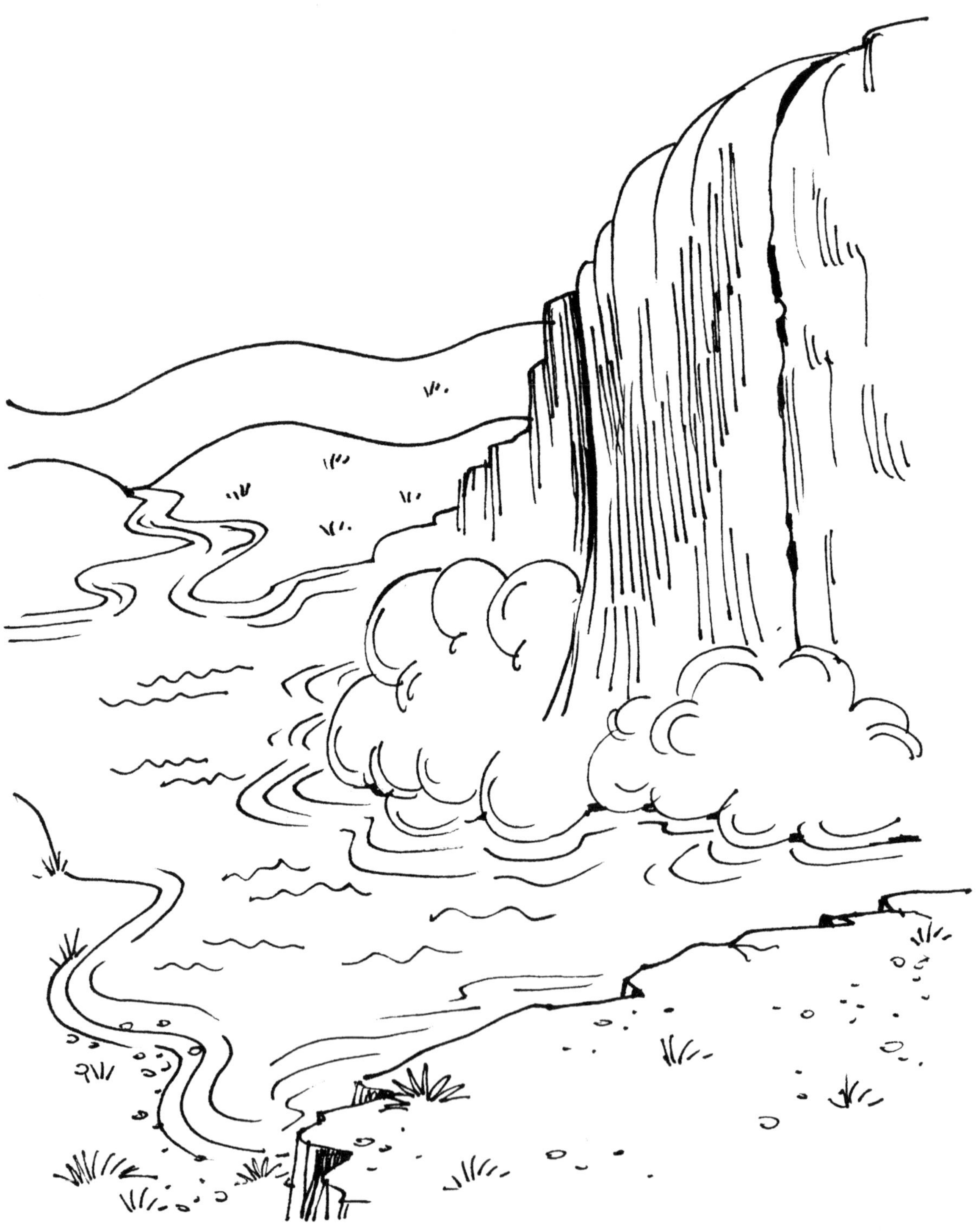

© 2001 *Thinking Publications.* Duplication permitted for educational use only.

Barrier Game Pieces

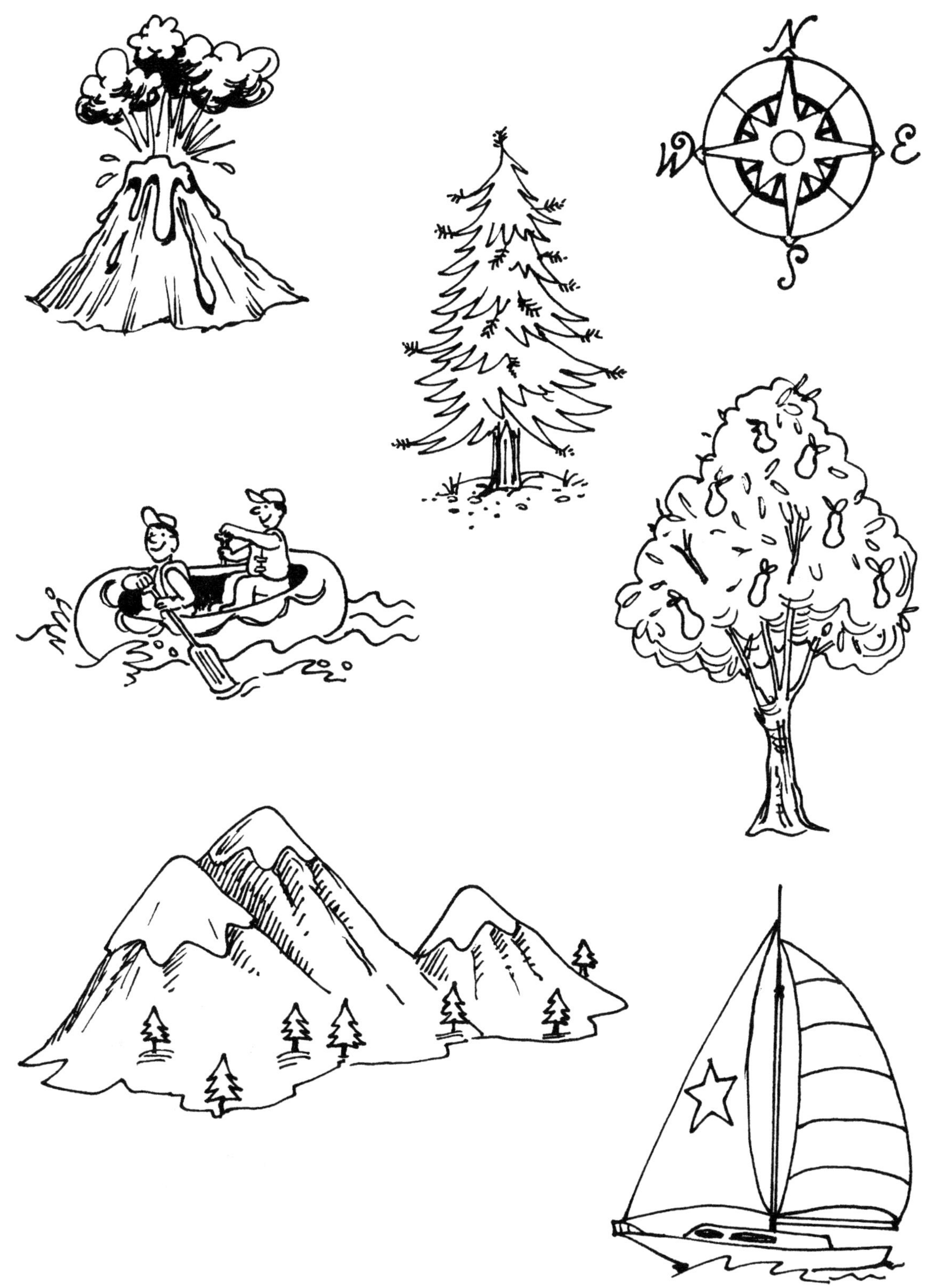

© 2001 *Thinking Publications.* Duplication permitted for educational use only.

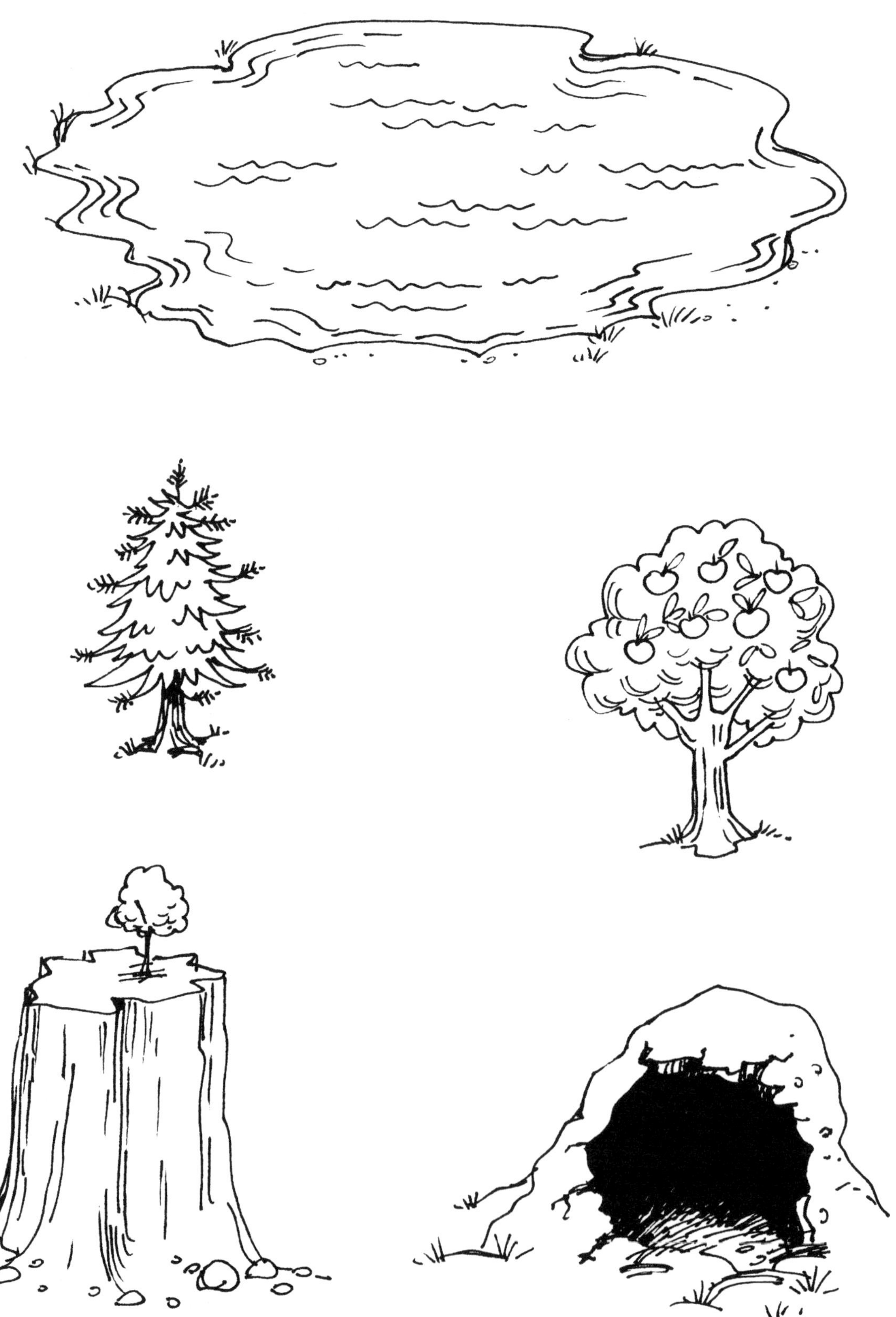

© 2001 *Thinking Publications.* Duplication permitted for educational use only.

Direction Strips

Put the pine tree on the west side
of the page, north of the river, and on the grass.

Put the tree near the waterfall.

Put the mountain range in the southwest corner.

Put the mountain range north of the river.

Put the raft in the river, halfway between
the large rock and the waterfall.

Put the raft in the lake.

Put the apple tree north of the river in the center, and put the
pear tree south of the river, just east of the large rock.

Put the apple tree next to another tree.

Put the volcano on the bottom.

Put the volcano north of the river and beside the waterfall.

© 2001 *Thinking Publications.* Duplication permitted for educational use only.

Put the cave north of the river, on the west side of the landscape, but touching the riverbank.

Put the cave near the rock.

Place the sailboat directly on top of the waterfall.

Put the sailboat sailing down the river.

Put the lake in the southeast corner of the landscape.

Put the lake beside the river.

Put the cliff south of the river, west of the rock, with the bottom of the cliff touching the grass.

Put the cliff touching the sky.

Put the small pine tree just to the left of the large rock.

Put the pear tree on top of the hill that faces the river.

© 2001 *Thinking Publications.* Duplication permitted for educational use only.

Rapid Write

HIT THE BULL'S-EYE (PART I)

Date: ______________________________

Name: ____

Directions

- My job is to write 3 directions using 3 objects.
- I'll need this paper, a pencil, the game board, and the game pieces.
- I'll know I'm finished when I have written 3 specific directions using complete sentences with correct punctuation.
- When I'm finished I'll share this work with the teacher.

Write 3 directions for placing 3 objects on the landscape.

1. ____

____

____

____

2. ____

____

____

____

3. ____

____

____

____

© 2001 *Thinking Publications.* Duplication permitted for educational use only.

HIT THE BULL'S-EYE: EVALUATING DIRECTIONS (PART II)

GOAL

To give and receive directions

BACKGROUND INFORMATION

In this lesson, students evaluate information and ask themselves the following questions: Does it make sense? Do I need more information? Is it a reasonable request? Students will apply the strategies they learned in *Part I* to a life skill (e.g., asking someone for directions, listing items needed and deciding where to acquire the items, and giving or following directions to a location).

OBJECTIVES

1. Ask for clarification when given insufficient information.
2. Use appropriate social language to gather information.
3. Draw conclusions about where different materials or information could be found.
4. Give clear and precise directions using specific vocabulary and reference points.

MATERIALS

1. *Community Map* (See page 67; duplicate and enlarge the graphic, color it, mount it onto construction paper or poster board, and laminate it for durability if desired. In addition to the large map, duplicate one map for each student.)
2. *Evaluate Directions to Hit the Bull's-Eye!* poster (Created earlier)
3. *Locate It Cards* (See pages 68–69; prepare one set for each pair of students; copy the cards onto heavy stock paper, cut them out, and laminate them for durability if desired.)
4. *Rapid Write: Hit the Bull's-Eye (Part II)* (See page 70; duplicate one per student.)

INTRODUCTION

Tie-in to Prior Learning

Remind students that in the last lesson *(Hit the Bull's-Eye: Evaluating Directions [Part I])* they practiced giving and receiving directions by listening, reading, speaking, or writing them. Tell students that in this lesson they will be using this skill in a more practical way.

Focus/Relevance

Ask students if they have ever moved into a new neighborhood, city, or state. Tell students that when you are new to an area you often have to ask for directions, such as where to go for the best shopping or places to eat. You may need to decide if the directions make sense and ask for clarification if they do not. Tell students that in this lesson they are all going to have an opportunity to both give clear directions and follow directions to find places within a community.

LESSON ACTIVITIES

1. Show students the large *Community Map*, and highlight various locations (e.g., the mall, the park, and the sports arena). Ask students how giving directions in a city might be different than giving directions using the game boards with land and water features from the previous lesson. Refer to the *Evaluate Directions to Hit the Bull's-Eye!* poster, reminding students to ask themselves the following questions when giving or receiving directions: Does the information make sense? Do I need more information (i.e., specific vocabulary, direction words, or reference points)? and Is it a reasonable request? Review the idea of using reference points, such as buildings, intersections, and street names, when giving directions.

2. Hand out a *Community Map* to each student. As a group, decide which direction on the map is north and have students draw a compass to help them remember. Tell students that they will take turns giving directions to the group to get to various locations on the map. The rest of the students will be the listeners. Whisper to the speaking student both the beginning and ending locations from one of the following examples:

   - The Bank to the Elementary School
   - The Post Office to the Mall
   - The Grocery Store to the Art Museum
   - The Library to the Water Tower
   - Willowbrook to the Hospital
   - The Art Museum to the High School

   The speaking student will then tell the rest of the class the starting point without telling the final destination. One listener may be at the front of a classroom pointing to the large map while other students follow along on their copy of the map. The listeners then follow the speaker's directions by tracing the route with their finger as if driving a car. Call on students to tell where their "cars" are parked after following all the directions. Check to be sure everyone has the same location. Discuss whether they "hit the bull's-eye" and if not, why.

3. Ask students to imagine that they have recently moved to this community and have signed up to play soccer. The coach has given each player a list of supplies that he or she will need to have before the first practice. Have students brainstorm places that might carry soccer or sporting supplies. Once students have named various stores that might carry sports equipment, ask how they might find the store. Elicit the idea of calling the store and asking for directions or asking a friend in the neighborhood for the best way to reach the store. Demonstrate how to use polite language when calling a store or asking a friend for directions (e.g., "Excuse me, I need some help finding Sports Town. Could you help me out?"). Remind students to indicate the starting point. Model writing directions quickly using abbreviations for directions and street names (Go N. on Park Ave. until you see the Elementary School on the corner of Park and Jupiter, then go E. one block to Preston) and checking for accuracy ("OK, just a minute, let me check to see if I've got this right"). Remind students that when they need to remember critical information, they need to "Take action! Write it down!"

4. Hand out the *Locate It Cards,* and have students work in pairs. Have one student be the new kid who asks where to find the item on the card and another student be the direction giver who gives the directions to find the item. Remind students to name a starting point and use reference points when appropriate. Have students all work in pairs simultaneously, or have one pair work while the rest of the class writes directions down as the direction giver is speaking.

5. Hand out the *Rapid Write: Hit the Bull's-Eye (Part II).* Read through the directions as a group and check for understanding. Ask students to write two sets of directions. Abbreviations are allowed if accuracy of the message is not effected. Remind students to reread for clarity before asking for help or finishing their work. Refer to the *Evaluate Directions to Hit the Bull's-Eye!* poster. Compare their responses and discuss.

CLOSURE

Summarize the lesson, review its relevance to students, and tie it to future learning. Congratulate students on demonstrating their use of two important life skills, both giving and following clear, precise directions. They have now practiced this skill both orally and in writing. In the next lesson *(Fact and Opinion: Persuading with Power [Part I]),* they will continue to improve their communication skills as they learn to distinguish fact statements and opinion statements.

Community Map

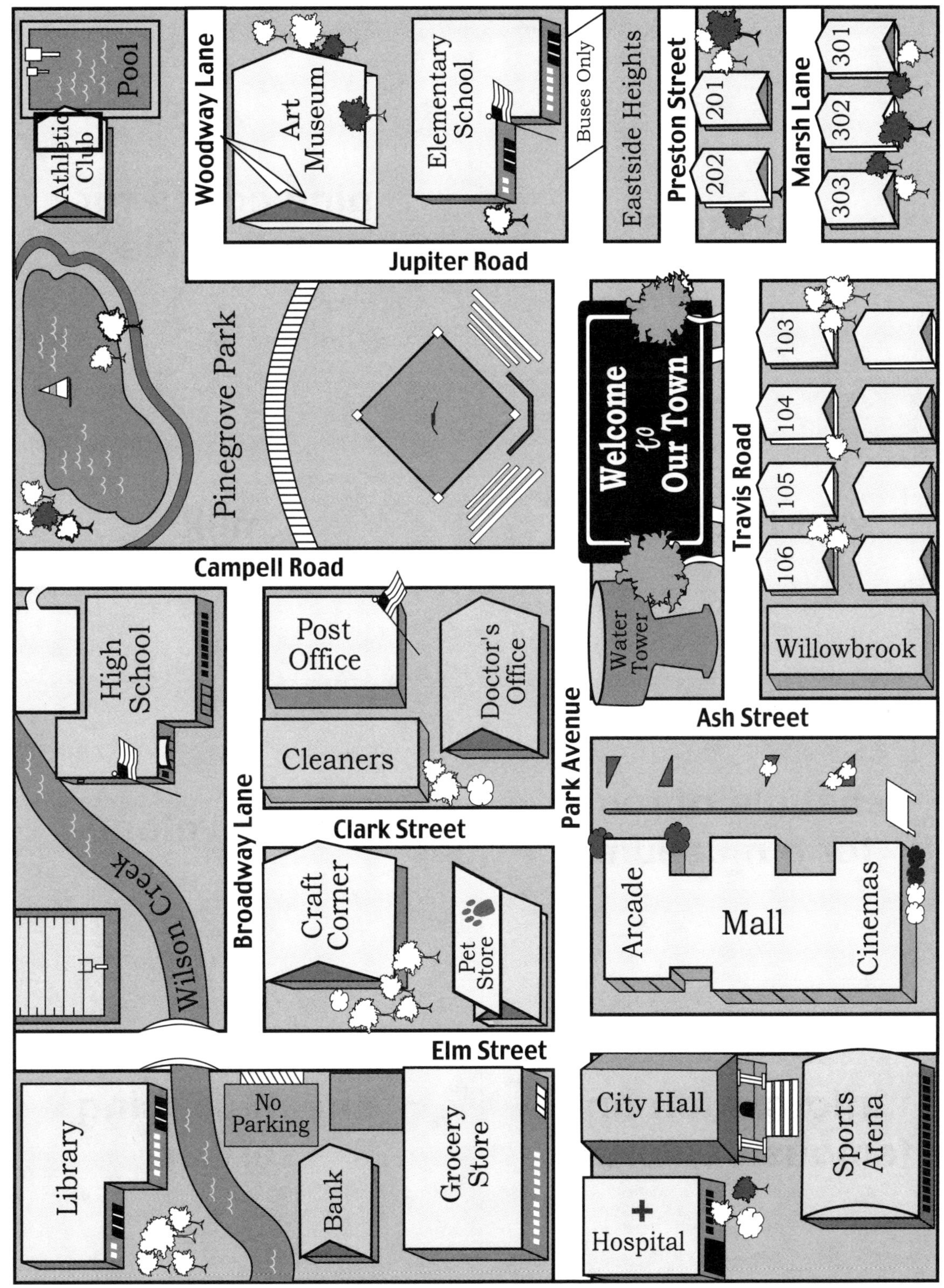

© 2001 *Thinking Publications.* Duplication permitted for educational use only.

Locate It Cards

sneakers	**pine cones for a craft project**
sports tickets	**milk**
schedule of tours for a museum	**large envelopes**
information on famous explorers	**check-cashing service**

© 2001 *Thinking Publications.* Duplication permitted for educational use only.

aerobic classes	video games
swim pass	pet vaccinations
bicycle permit	movie schedule
dry cleaning	library books

© 2001 *Thinking Publications.* Duplication permitted for educational use only.

RAPID WRITE

HIT THE BULL'S-EYE (PART II)

Date: ____________________________

Name: ____

Directions

- My job is to write 2 sets of directions using abbreviations for directions and street names.
- I'll need this paper, a pencil, and the *Community Map.*
- I'll know I'm finished when I have written specific directions using complete sentences with correct punctuation.
- When I'm finished I'll share this work with the teacher.

Use the *Community Map to* write directions.

- **Directions from 104 Travis Road to the Pool:**

- **Directions from the east end of Pinegrove Park to the Hospital**

© 2001 *Thinking Publications.* Duplication permitted for educational use only.

FACT AND OPINION: PERSUADING WITH POWER (PART I)

GOAL

To differentiate fact from opinion

BACKGROUND INFORMATION

The purpose of this lesson is to help students distinguish fact statements from opinion statements, which is an evaluative listening skill. Learning the difference between fact and opinion allows students to use better descriptive language. For example, when describing, students can use specific and factual language, such as "The apple is red and has seeds," and express an opinion, such as "The apple tastes good."

Part I will teach students to use fact statements and opinion statements to persuade a listener to share a particular point of view. As students reach their later elementary years, they are further expected to be able to write a persuasive paragraph, which is the focus of *Part II*.

OBJECTIVES

1. Recognize keywords that identify fact and opinion statements.
2. Write fact statements and opinion statements using keywords.

MATERIALS

1. *Use Facts and Opinions to Persuade!* graphic (See page 74; duplicate and enlarge the graphic, color it, mount it onto construction paper or poster board, and laminate it for durability if desired.)
2. Advertisements (Cut from magazines or newspapers.)
3. *Rapid Write: Fact and Opinion (Part I)* (See page 75; duplicate one per group.)

INTRODUCTION

Tie-in to Prior Learning

Review the skills learned in the *Hit the Bull's-Eye: Evaluating Directions* lessons regarding giving and receiving clear and precise directions, evaluating information, and requesting clarification when necessary. Ask students whether the directions included more facts or more opinions. Elicit the idea that when giving and receiving directions, facts must be used. Explain that in this lesson they will learn about using both facts and opinions to persuade others.

Focus/Relevance

1. Ask students if they ever watch television. If so, what is the information that the television provides during and between shows? Elicit the idea of commercials. Tell students that today you have a special commercial to share with them. Read the following script:

   Attention students! In our lunchroom just for today you will have the opportunity to try a brand new treat from our south-of-the-border neighbor, Mexico. This delectable treat comes in a beautiful shade of brown. It is sweet, nutty, and comes in different shapes. It is a delicious praline. It's the best snack you'll ever find. It is available only during lunch today. It is free with the purchase of the regular school lunch. Don't be left out! Buy your lunch ticket now!

2. Ask students if this commercial tempted them to spend their hard-earned snack money on a praline instead of another snack. Tell students that in this lesson they will be talking about the use of fact statements and opinion statements to persuade their listeners to buy a special product, just like an advertiser uses a mix of facts and opinions to persuade consumers.

LESSON ACTIVITIES

1. Show the *Use Facts and Opinions to Persuade!* poster. Read and discuss the difference between factual information that can be proven true and opinion words that show a perspective or point of view about something. Compare the two people in the poster; when they think differently, they are apart; when they use facts and opinions to persuade each other, they meet in the middle. Discuss what makes a statement factual. Elicit ways to prove a statement is fact by checking an encyclopedia, using the Internet, looking in resource books, or asking knowledgeable people. Discuss how factual information can be checked by seeing it for ourselves. Have students brainstorm words and phrases that signal opinion statements (e.g., *like, don't like, good, bad,* or *I think*). Read the praline advertisement again, and ask students to identify factual information and words that signal opinions.

2. Share examples of advertisements from magazines or newspapers. Analyze the facts and opinions in the ads. Then tell students that they have been given an important job as an advertiser for a major company; they are going to work with a creative team to write a commercial for a product that has to do with a holiday (e.g., holiday decorations, Halloween costumes or candy, or Valentine's Day cards). Divide students into small teams of two or three. Tell students that each team will be responsible for writing at least two factual statements about the product, for writing at least two opinion statements, and for drawing an illustration to look at or show during the commercial. Remind students to use catchy phrases for both their facts and opinions.

3. Model the process for the group. Choose a product (e.g., Prouty's Pumpkin Patch). Let students share factual information that should be included in the commercial such as the location, price, hours, and phone number. List several of these ideas. Then have students brainstorm opinion statements that can make the commercial more appealing to a consumer, such as "The best pumpkins in town are at Prouty's!" or "Every home should have one pumpkin for each family member!" Tell students that there is an immediate deadline for the completion of their advertisement so they must work quickly.
4. Hand out *Rapid Write: Fact and Opinion (Part I)*. Read through the directions as a group and check for understanding. Ask students to write two fact statements and two opinion statements for the team's commercial. Tell them to draw their illustration on a separate sheet of paper. Remind students to reread for clarity before asking for help or finishing their work. Discuss their responses.

   HINT: A fun way to expand this lesson is to allow students to record their commercial announcements on audiotape or videotape.

5. Let each team share its commercial with the group. Have the other teams identify the fact and opinion statements. Allow students to offer compliments to each creative team.

CLOSURE

Summarize the lesson, review its relevance to students, and tie it to future learning. Compliment students for their creative use of facts and opinions in writing commercials. Tell them that in the next lesson *(Fact and Opinion: Persuading with Power [Part II])* they will be using fact and opinion statements in writing as a way to persuade a listener to consider their point of view.

Use Facts and Opinions to Persuade!

A **FACT** has a clue to **PROVE** it is true.

An **OPINION** shows your **POINT OF VIEW.**

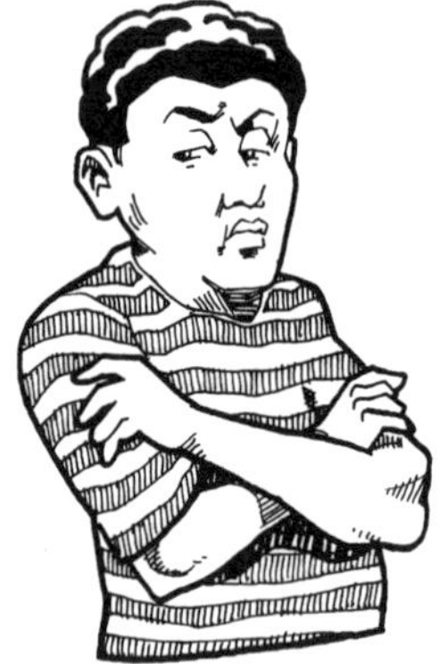

He thinks...

Persuade

Convince
Sway
Debate
Argue points
Change a point of view

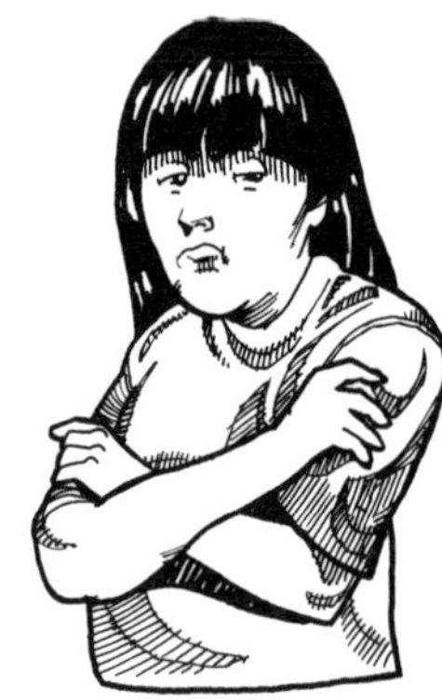

I think...

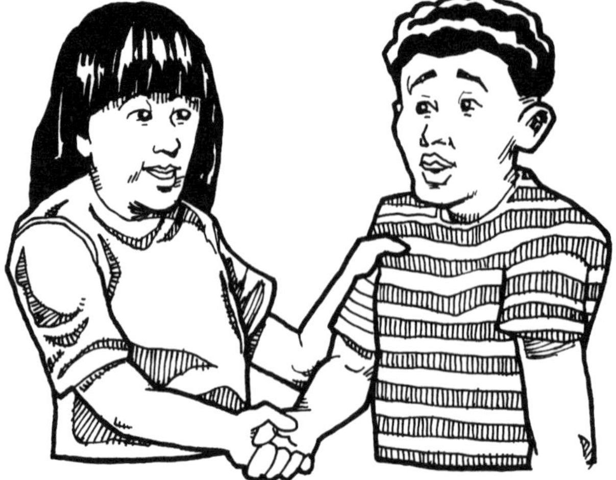

We think...

© 2001 *Thinking Publications.* Duplication permitted for educational use only.

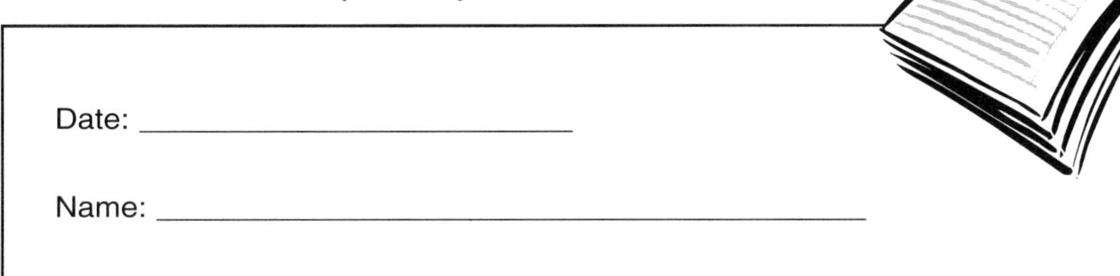

RAPID WRITE

FACT AND OPINION (PART I)

Date: ______________________________

Name: ____

Directions

- Our job is to write 2 fact statements and 2 opinion statements about our product. Then we'll draw an illustration of the product on a separate sheet of paper.
- We'll need this paper, a blank sheet of paper, and a pencil.
- We'll know we're finished when we have 4 complete sentences with correct punctuation and an illustration.
- When we're finished we'll share this work with the teacher.

Write your script for a commercial.

Product: ____

Fact: ____

____

Fact: ____

____

Opinion: ____

____

Opinion: ____

____

Draw you illustration on a separate sheet of paper.

© 2001 *Thinking Publications.* Duplication permitted for educational use only.

FACT AND OPINION: PERSUADING WITH POWER (PART II)

GOAL

To differentiate fact from opinion

BACKGROUND INFORMATION

The purpose of this lesson is to help students generate fact statements and opinion statements when they write a persuasive paragraph. Learning the difference between fact and opinion allows students to use better descriptive language. For example, when describing, students can use specific and factual language, such as "The apple is red and has seeds," and express an opinion, such as "The apple tastes good."

In *Part I*, students used fact statements and opinion statements to persuade a listener to share a particular point of view in a simple commercial. In this lesson, they will take this knowledge to a higher level as they apply the strategy to personal and academic writing activities.

OBJECTIVES

1. Generate fact statements and opinion statements using keywords.
2. Write fact statements and opinion statements to make a persuasive argument.
3. Generate a concluding statement that summarizes a persuasive position.

MATERIALS

1. *Use Facts and Opinions to Persuade!* poster (Created earlier)
2. *Rapid Write: Fact and Opinion (Part II)* (See page 79; duplicate one per student.)
3. *Just Do It! Review Activity One* (See page 80; duplicate one per student.)
4. Unit One posters (Created earlier)

INTRODUCTION

Tie-in to Prior Learning

Review the *Use Facts and Opinions to Persuade!* poster. Have students recall examples of fact statements and opinion statements that they used in their commercials from the last lesson *(Part I)*. Review some of the keywords that help to differentiate fact from opinion. Explain that in this lesson they will use persuasion to try to convince fellow classmates to adopt another point of view.

Focus/Relevance

Tell students about a news feature you saw recently. In this news report, people were trying to persuade their neighbors to join them in volunteering to clean up the neighborhood park. Explain that you wanted to help but just did not know how to get started. The people on the news used a strategy to help convince the neighbors to join in this project. Tell students that this lesson will help them practice a strategy for persuading others and they will also learn to recognize when they are being persuaded.

LESSON ACTIVITIES

1. Refer to the *Use Facts and Opinions to Persuade!* poster, and explain that using fact statements and opinion statements is helpful when trying to persuade someone to share your point of view. The strategy for persuasion requires that the speaker think about the listener's perspective or point of view. Refer back to the news story about neighborhood cleanup. Ask students why the neighbors might not want to help clean up the neighborhood. Discuss what their arguments against helping might be (e.g., "I do not have time," "'The other guy' will take care of it," or "I do not want to be in charge"). Now discuss the arguments for helping (e.g., "If we all work together, it will take less time;" "One person cannot do it alone;" and "Everyone will share the benefits of having a beautiful neighborhood park"). Tell students that when trying to persuade someone to share a point of view they must use ideas that include both facts and opinions.

2. Divide students into pairs and tell them that they will be debating for and against a topic. Each member of the pair will have to give two facts and two opinions to support his or her assigned position. Model the use of phrases, such as "I think that..." or "Everyone should...," as a way to share an opinion. Discuss the concept of including a concluding statement (e.g., "So let's go clean up the park today!") as a way to finish their turn in a persuasive discussion and summarize their position. Have students pick one of the topics from the list below. Choose who will be arguing for and who against each topic. Remind students they may have to take on the perspective of an opposing view (e.g., be the teacher when arguing in favor of homework). Ask students to identify which statements are fact and which are opinion as they listen to the different arguments. Some topics may include:

   - Having homework
   - Adding fast food to the school lunch menu
   - Having a monkey as a pet
   - Doing exercise
   - Having more computer time at school

- Having your own TV in your bedroom
- Having your own phone in your bedroom
- Staying up until midnight
- Having friends over on a school night

3. Hand out *Rapid Write: Fact and Opinion (Part II)*. Read through the directions as a group and check for understanding. Tell students that they will be writing a letter to a family member about something students want. Have students share their ideas about what they might want. Remind students to reread for clarity before asking for help or finishing their work. Discuss their responses.

   To generalize to academic goals, ask students what they would need to add to what they have written if they were writing a complete persuasive paper. Elicit the concepts of topic sentences, supporting fact or opinion statements, and conclusions.

CLOSURE

Summarize the lesson, review its relevance to students, and tie it to future learning. Remind students that facts and opinions are essential when trying to persuade someone else to believe their point of view. Explain that they also need to try to predict the point of view or potential argument of the listener, so they can decide which facts and which opinions will be most effective. Tell students that in the next lessons (Unit Two) they will begin to think about their word power.

JUST DO IT!

Hand out *Just Do It! Review Activity One.* Explain that this is a homework activity that reviews the lessons from Unit One. Refer to the previously created Unit One posters. Briefly review vocabulary from the posters. Review the directions for *Just Do It! Review Activity One.* Set a due date for the assignment.

Rapid Write

FACT AND OPINION (PART II)

Date: ____________________________

Name: ____

Directions

- My job is to write a persuasive letter to a family member about something I want.
- I'll need this paper and a pencil.
- I'll know I'm finished when I have included an introduction, 2 facts, 2 opinions, a conclusion, and an action statement all written in complete sentences with correct punctuation.
- When I'm finished I'll share this work with the teacher.

Write a persuasive letter about something you want.

(Greeting) Dear ________________,

(Introduction) I think we should ____________________

____

(Body) ____________________________________

- 2 facts ____________________________________

____

- 2 opinions ____________________________________

____

(Conclusion) ____________________________________

____

(Action statement) So, let's ____________________ today!

Love,

© 2001 *Thinking Publications.* Duplication permitted for educational use only.

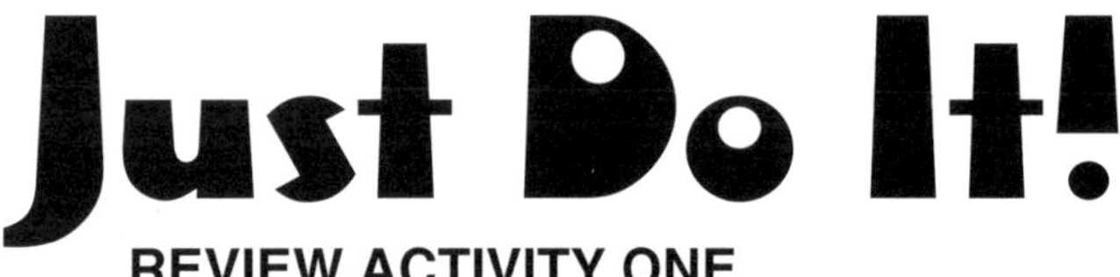

REVIEW ACTIVITY ONE

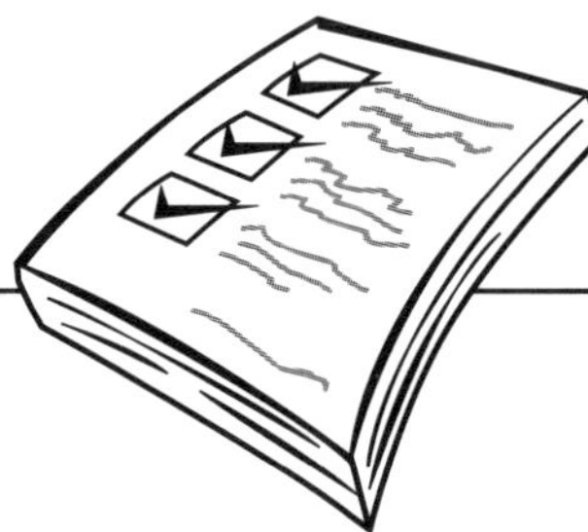

Complete the following tasks with a family member.
Initial each after you've completed it.

_____ Explain the difference between critical and noncritical information.

_____ Tell 2 critical pieces of information you should get when taking a telephone message.

_____ Watch the news tonight. Listen for 1 news segment that is relevant to you or your family and 1 news segment that is irrelevant. Write the topics in the spaces below.

Relevant segment: ________________________________

Irrelevant segment: ________________________________

_____ Practice giving directions between 2 places. Record the 2 places below.

From: ______________________________

To: ________________________________

_____ Have a family member give you directions. Practice writing directions using abbreviations and asking for clarification if needed.

_____ Try to persuade a family member to take you to a fast-food restaurant of your choice. Be sure to include 2 fact statements and 2 opinion statements.

Student signature ____

Family member signature __________________________________

This review activity is due back at school on:

© 2001 *Thinking Publications.* Duplication permitted for educational use only.

UNIT TWO

GOAL-SETTING ACTIVITY TWO

GOAL

To encourage self-improvement through goal setting

BACKGROUND INFORMATION

The purpose of this lesson is to help students learn the steps for setting and meeting a goal (i.e., identifying a need, formulating a goal, practicing the steps to reach the goal, revising the goal as needed, and evaluating progress) and apply the steps to setting goals for building vocabulary and word power. Rather than expecting students to set goals independently, the goal-setting process is modeled. Writing a goal for word power could be teacher directed, but reflection on the need for the goal and how the goal might be useful will be individual for each student since each student's use of the goal is different.

OBJECTIVES

1. Understand the following goal-setting concepts: achieving a goal, revising a goal, and evaluating progress.
2. Evaluate progress on achieving the previous goal.
3. Tell how the previous goal was met.
4. Write a goal related to improving word power and identify when this skill is important at home, at school, and in the community.

MATERIALS

1. Unit One posters
2. *Goal Setting: Activity One* (Each student's previously completed goal sheet.)
3. *Goal Setting: Activity Two* (See page 86; duplicate one per student.)

INTRODUCTION

Tie-in to Prior Learning

Compliment students on their hard work during Unit One to improve their skill at being effective listeners. Remind students that in *Goal-Setting Activity One* they set a specific goal that could be focused on for improvement. Refer to posters from Unit One, and use them for discussion while completing activities in this lesson.

Focus/Relevance

1. Write the word *evaluate* where everyone can see it. Brainstorm various ways to evaluate something (e.g., watching replays after a football game or having a listener offer tips after hearing your speech). Review the concept of using evaluation as a tool to decide whether students have successfully completed their goals.

2. Tell students that learning is easier when goals are set and steps for achieving them are planned. Remind them that achieving a goal requires a strategy—or a standard way of attacking a problem. Setting goals can help students achieve many different skills at home, at school, and in the community. Tell students that it is time to evaluate their progress on the strategies learned in Unit One.

LESSON ACTIVITIES

1. Hand out each student's copy of *Goal Setting: Activity One.* Refer to each of the Unit One posters. Encourage students to reflect on the steps they took to achieve the goal written on their goal sheet as well as how the goal has been helpful at home, in school, or in the community. Remind students that they will want to continue to practice each completed goal while targeting a new one.

2. Give each student a copy of *Goal Setting: Activity Two.* Remind students that in the previous unit they practiced an important communication goal by learning to be better listeners. Explain to students that in this unit they will be learning ways to communicate in many different situations. Expand on this concept by discussing the word *communication* and what it means to be an effective communicator. Elicit ideas, such as being able to learn information, take messages, write for work or pleasure, or know what to say when conversing with peers or adults. Expand on the concept of being a good communicator by discussing a few examples of how communication styles change depending on the situation (e.g., talking to an infant versus talking with a principal). Explain that in this unit students will learn ways to consider the situation when deciding on their choice of words.

3. Write the words *word power* where everyone can see them. Write the following goal where everyone can see it:

   I will choose powerful words that fit the situation to express my ideas.

   Tell students that this will be their main goal in this unit. Explain that *powerful* means clear and precise and that the words they choose to say a message can change with the situation.

Tell students that they will learn more about how to use powerful words in every situation in the lessons to follow.

4. Read through *Goal Setting: Activity Two* as a group and check for understanding. Have students complete the goal statement on their goal sheet by adding the words *powerful* and *situation*. Tell students to write examples of when they think using powerful words is important at home, at school, and in the community. Remind students to reread for clarity before asking for help or finishing their work. Discuss their responses.

   HINT: If students have difficulty generating situations, use one of the following ideas:
   An example of when a goal is important

   - at home is when you need to explain why you are late.
   - at school is when you need to write about why a historical event happened.
   - in the community is when you need to give directions to a restaurant to someone.

CLOSURE

Summarize the lesson, review its relevance to students, and tie it to future learning. Recap for students by explaining that they have set an important goal and in the next lesson they will begin working on the first step to achieve their goal. Have them sign and date *Goal Setting: Activity Two.* By signing and dating the goal sheet, they are promising to concentrate and work on the goal. Explain that you will also sign their goal sheets as a promise to help each student reach his or her goal. Encourage students to take the goal sheet home to share with their family, but request that they return it by a set time with a family member's initials. Keep the goal sheets for future reference as they will be used again during the next goal-setting lesson (*Goal-Setting Activity Three*). When the goal sheets are returned, you might want to keep them all in one folder or create a separate folder for each student.

HINT: Offer a tangible or social reward for returning the goal sheet with a family member's initials.

GOAL SETTING

ACTIVITY TWO

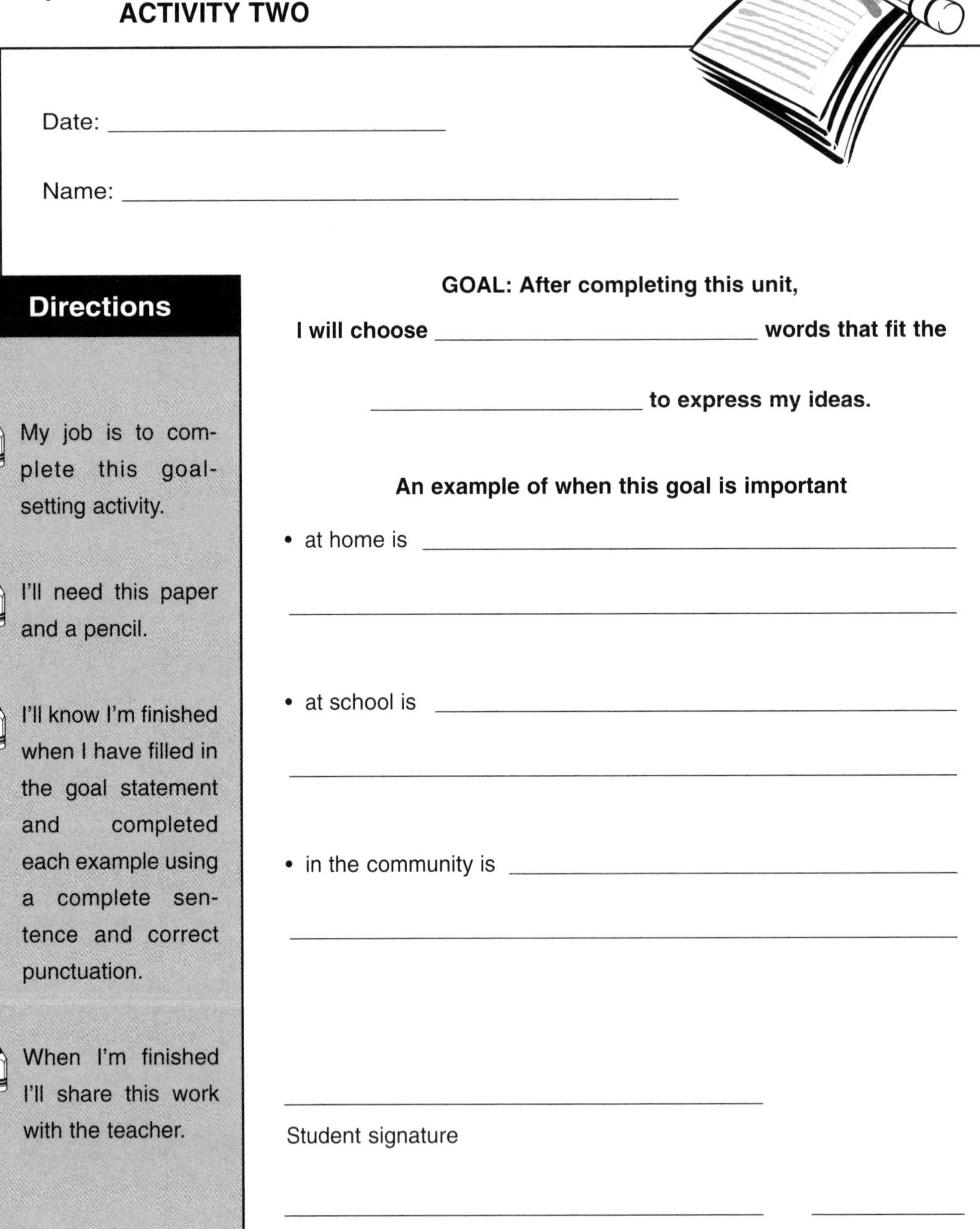

Date: ______________________

Name: ______________________

Directions

- My job is to complete this goal-setting activity.
- I'll need this paper and a pencil.
- I'll know I'm finished when I have filled in the goal statement and completed each example using a complete sentence and correct punctuation.
- When I'm finished I'll share this work with the teacher.

GOAL: After completing this unit,

I will choose ______________ words that fit the

______________ to express my ideas.

An example of when this goal is important

- at home is ______________________

____

- at school is ______________________

____

- in the community is ______________________

____

____
Student signature

____
Teacher signature

____
Family member initials

© 2001 *Thinking Publications.* Duplication permitted for educational use only.

CODE-SWITCHING TOOLS: INTRODUCING COMMUNICATION REGISTERS

GOAL

To identify and switch between communication registers

BACKGROUND INFORMATION

The purpose of this lesson is to introduce students to the concept of changing communication registers (i.e., changing language to fit a situation) to accomplish a variety of communication tasks. In this lesson, the three communication registers—social language (e.g., talking with friends), work/school/community language (e.g., asking a teacher a question), and written language (e.g., typing a book report)—will be introduced. The subsequent three lessons will each highlight a grammatical form (i.e., subject/verb, adverbs/adjectives, and synonyms) that makes changing a communication register possible. Students will learn the term *code-switching,* which refers to switching a communication register to fit the situation (i.e., location, person, and activity). Many students must be explicitly taught that they need to switch communication registers as it makes a huge impact on how students are perceived by their listeners, especially teachers and authority figures. Students' school and work success is highly dependent on their level of flexibility when making these language decisions (Payne, 1998). This lesson strengthens metalinguistic skills, such as flexible use of vocabulary in both oral and written language relating to communication registers.

OBJECTIVES

1. Identify three communication registers: social, work/school/community, and written language.
2. Recognize the need to shift communication register according to the situation (i.e., location, person, and activity).
3. Shift communication registers from social language to work/school/community language and written language.

MATERIALS

1. *Use Word Power to Code Switch!* graphic (See page 90; duplicate and enlarge the graphic, color it, mount it onto construction paper or poster board, and laminate it for durability if desired.)

2. *Code-Switching Cartoons* graphics (See pages 91–93; duplicate and enlarge each cartoon, color it, mount it onto construction paper or poster board, and laminate it for durability if desired.)

3. *Rhinos Who Snowboard* (1997) by Julie Mammano (This book was selected because it contains a

good example of social language, the topic of snowboarding is interesting to students, it includes higher level vocabulary, and the glossary of terms translates the social language to more formal language. Any book with similar characteristics can be substituted.)

4. *Rapid Write: Code-Switching Tools One* (See page 94; duplicate one per student.)

INTRODUCTION

Tie-in to Prior Learning

Remind students that in *Goal-Setting Activity Two* they wrote a new goal that will help them become more effective communicators. Tell students that in this lesson they will discover how they can use powerful words and language in different ways when talking and writing.

Focus/Relevance

Ask students what they plan to do after they graduate from school. Would they like to work at an important job? Stress that being able to code switch or play the "language game" ensures that they will "win" at school with better grades, "win" in the job market by being able to find good jobs, and "win" with their friends because they will be more powerful communicators.

HINT: If you are feeling dramatic, enter the room in secret agent character (e.g., wearing dark sunglasses and a trench coat with "Mission Impossible" music playing). Begin the lesson by issuing the statement: "Welcome ___ graders. Your mission, should you choose to accept it, is to use word power to code switch!"

LESSON ACTIVITIES

1. Show the *Use Word Power to Code Switch!* poster. Read through each section and highlight its components. Emphasize that the language used to communicate can be very informal and social with family, friends, and people who are very familiar; it can be more formal with authority figures, acquaintances, or unfamiliar people in a work, school, or community situation; or it can be formal for written language, which is carefully planned communication that follows grammatical rules. Students, like the detective on the poster, must "crack the code" and decide on the most appropriate type of language for the situation. Discuss how they crack the code by considering the location, the person, and the activity. Remind students that they must make a decision about the best choice of language—the code—as they begin a conversation and be ready to code switch as the situation changes. Point out the arrow, which symbolizes switching codes.

2. Show the *Code-Switching Cartoons* posters. Read the *Code-Switching Cartoon One* poster, which depicts several boys riding skateboards and talking about skateboarding. Discuss the language

being used by the boys in the cartoon and decide which code the boys are using. Point out that the boys are using the term *aggro* to mean *fearless, phat* to mean *really big,* and *ollie* to mean a *maneuver.* Ask students to name similar terms they might use with their friends. Ask students to speculate about what the boys are getting ready to do (i.e., ask Mrs. Rodriguez a question). Refer to the *Use Word Power to Code Switch!* poster again, and encourage students to consider whether they think the boys will need to code switch before talking to Mrs. Rodriguez. Ask what they think Mrs. Rodriguez would think if they do not switch codes. Refer to the poster and review the area for work/school/community language (i.e., make careful word choices when talking to authority figures, acquaintances, or unfamiliar people). Read the *Code-Switching Cartoon Two* poster, which depicts two students approaching Mrs. Rodriguez with a question. Point out the "code switch" of "Yo! Cody has an awesome board!" to "Good morning, Mrs. Rodriguez. Do you have time for a question?" Continue to highlight the code switch from the first cartoon to the second cartoon.

3. Lead a similar discussion of *Code-Switching Cartoon Three.* Refer to the first cartoon that uses, "Yo!" instead of "Hello!" Ask students to share other kinds of greetings (e.g., shaking hands, waving, saluting, or using a greeting in a letter). Compare the following terms: "Yo" is very informal, like wearing shorts; "Hello" is a little more dressed up like wearing nice pants or a skirt; and a written greeting like "Dear Sir" is fancy, like a tuxedo or ball gown. Remind students that written language is the most formal language; it has strict grammatical rules that need to be considered. Written language requires planning and prewriting. Point out that as Cody writes his article he plans and prewrites.

4. Read *Rhinos Who Snowboard.* Have students decide the book's code and then practice translating the code to work/school/community language as you read the book.

5. Hand out *Rapid Write: Code-Switching Tools One*. Read through the directions as a group and check for understanding. Ask students to change each statement from social language to work/school/community language. Remind students to reread for clarity before asking for help or finishing their work. Work through this activity as a group or have students work independently. Discuss their responses.

CLOSURE

Summarize the lesson, review its relevance to students, and tie it to future learning. Tell students that they have learned a powerful tool in this lesson. Briefly discuss why recognizing the need to code switch and use the right words for location, person, or activity can be valuable for their success. Tell students that in the next lesson *(Code-Switching Tools: Identifying Subjects and Verbs)* they will continue to discover powerful language tools.

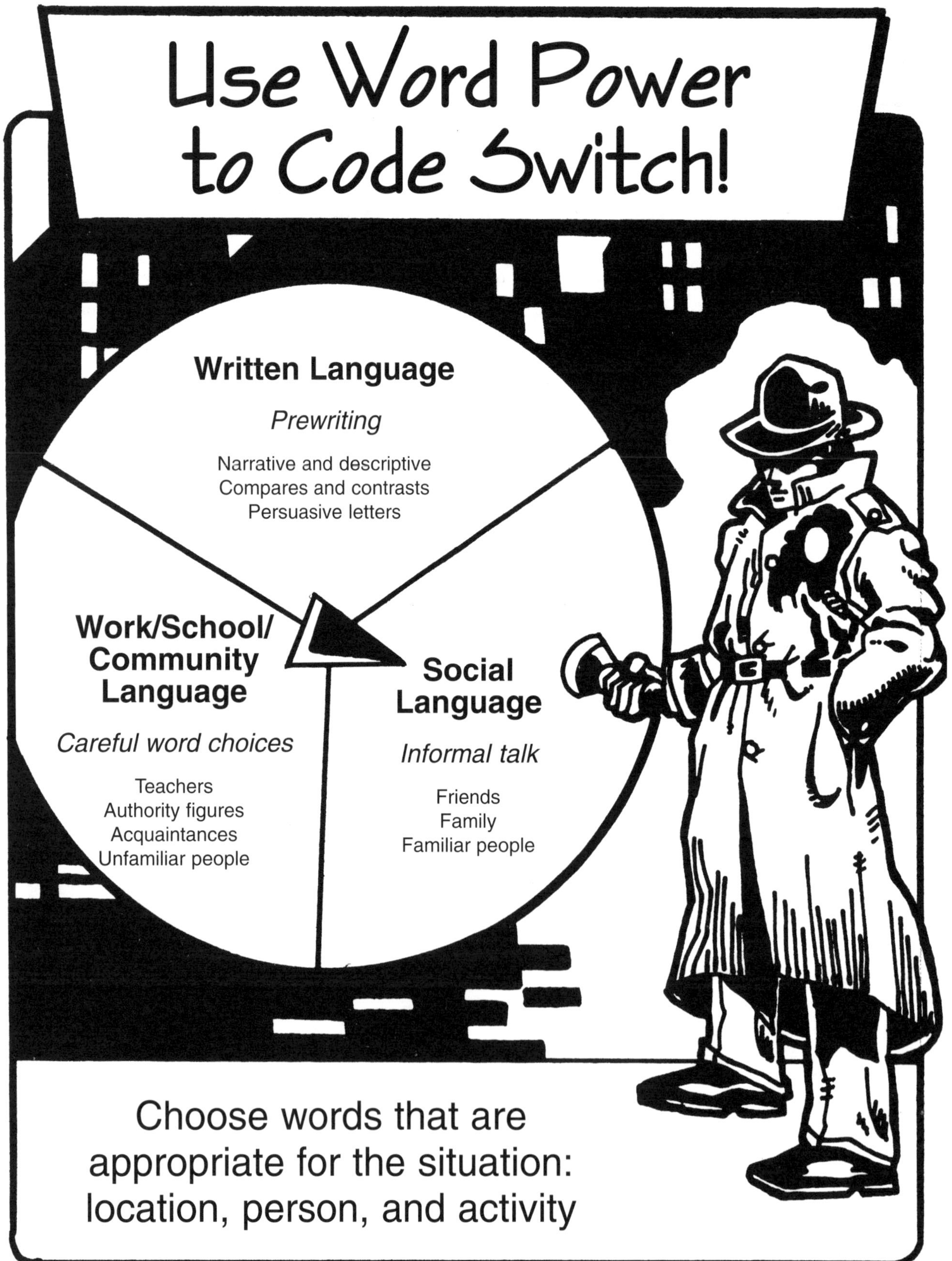

© 2001 *Thinking Publications.* Duplication permitted for educational use only.

Code-Switching Cartoon One

Yo! Cody has an awesome board! He's a radical spin master. Totally catches phat air when he ollies!
Yeah! His board has a slick deck. Radical colors too. I could go totally aggro with a board like that!
I heard he won it in some kind of contest. Let's check it out with Mrs. Rodriguez.

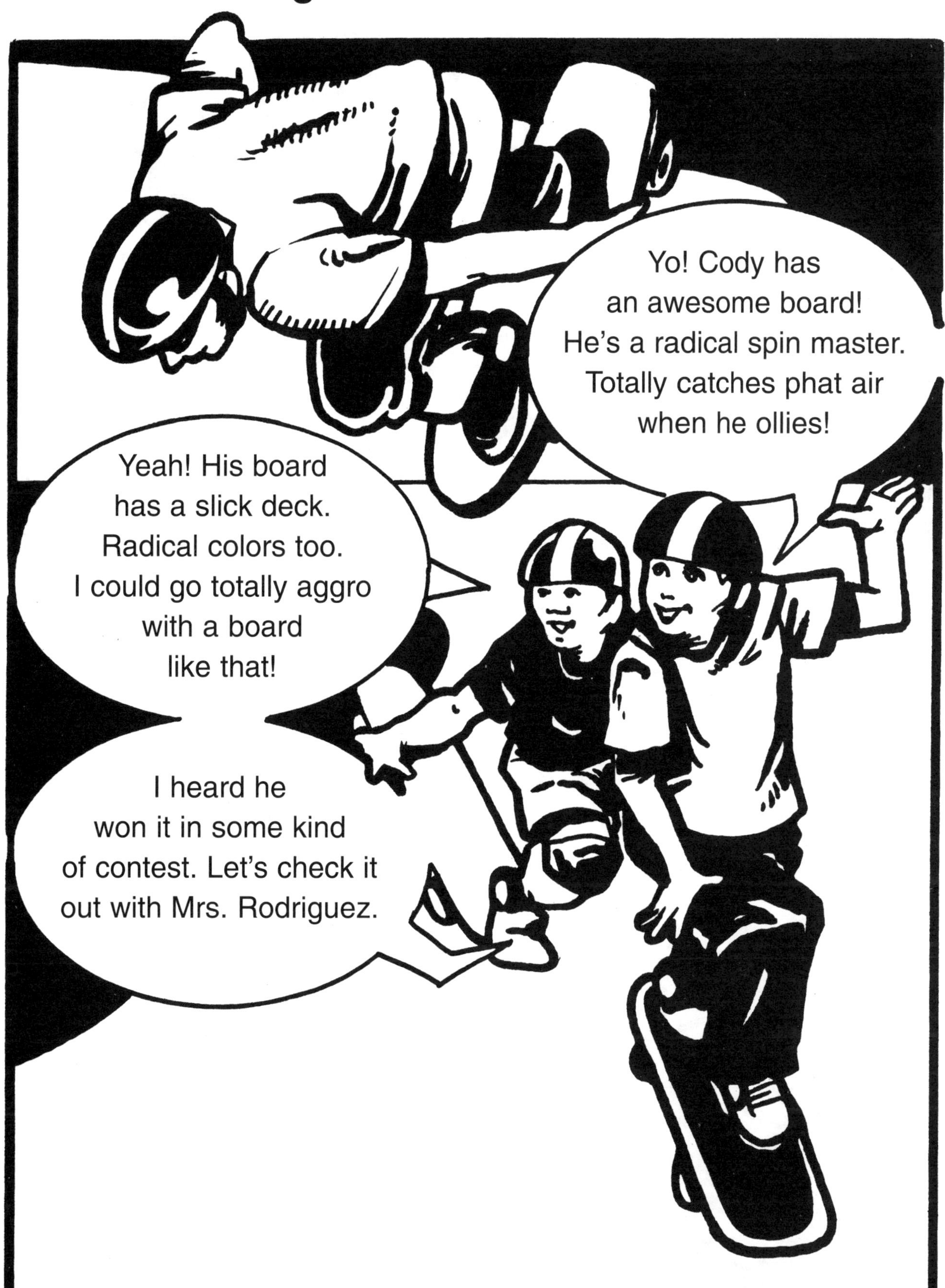

© 2001 *Thinking Publications.* Duplication permitted for educational use only.

Code-Switching Cartoon Two

Good morning, Mrs. Rodriguez. Do you have time for a question? We really like Cody's skateboard! He knows tricks to make it spin around, and he can jump very high with it!
We heard he won it in some kind of contest and wanted to ask if you knew about anything like that.
I've seen his skateboard. It has custom-made wheels and it's plastic rather than wooden. It's decorated with bright colors too. I could learn a lot of tricks with a board like that!
Your description sounds like a great article for the descriptive writing contest in the local paper. You might win enough money to buy one!

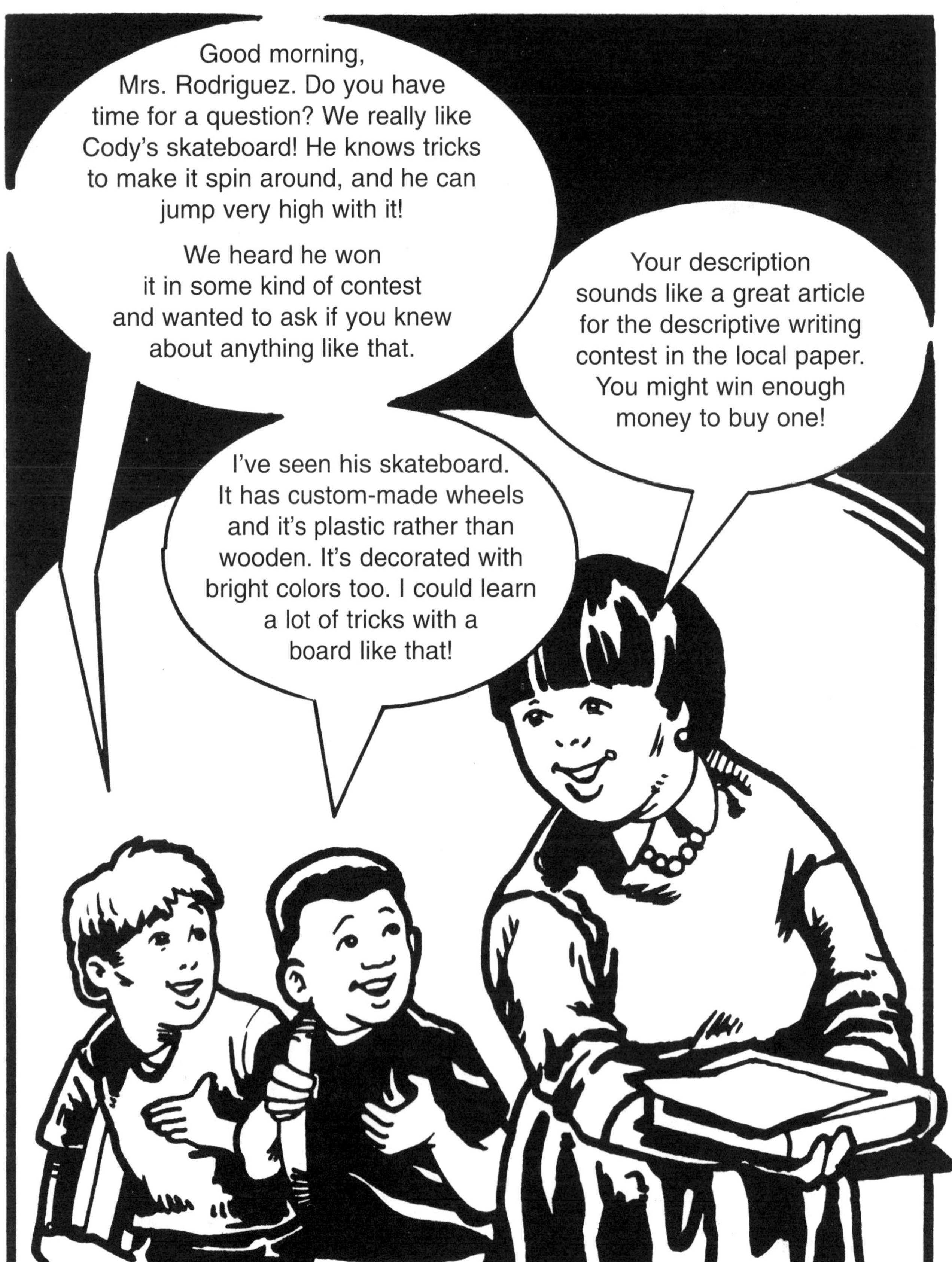

© 2001 *Thinking Publications.* Duplication permitted for educational use only.

Code-Switching Cartoon Three

Plan
I need to have a topic paragraph.
I will add descriptive details.
I must remember a concluding paragraph.
Prewrite
It is extremely important to consider several features when selecting a skateboard! Shoppers need to be aware of how each feature will effect performance as it pertains to the skill level of the rider. Size, shape, composition, and decorations are key to choosing the right board.

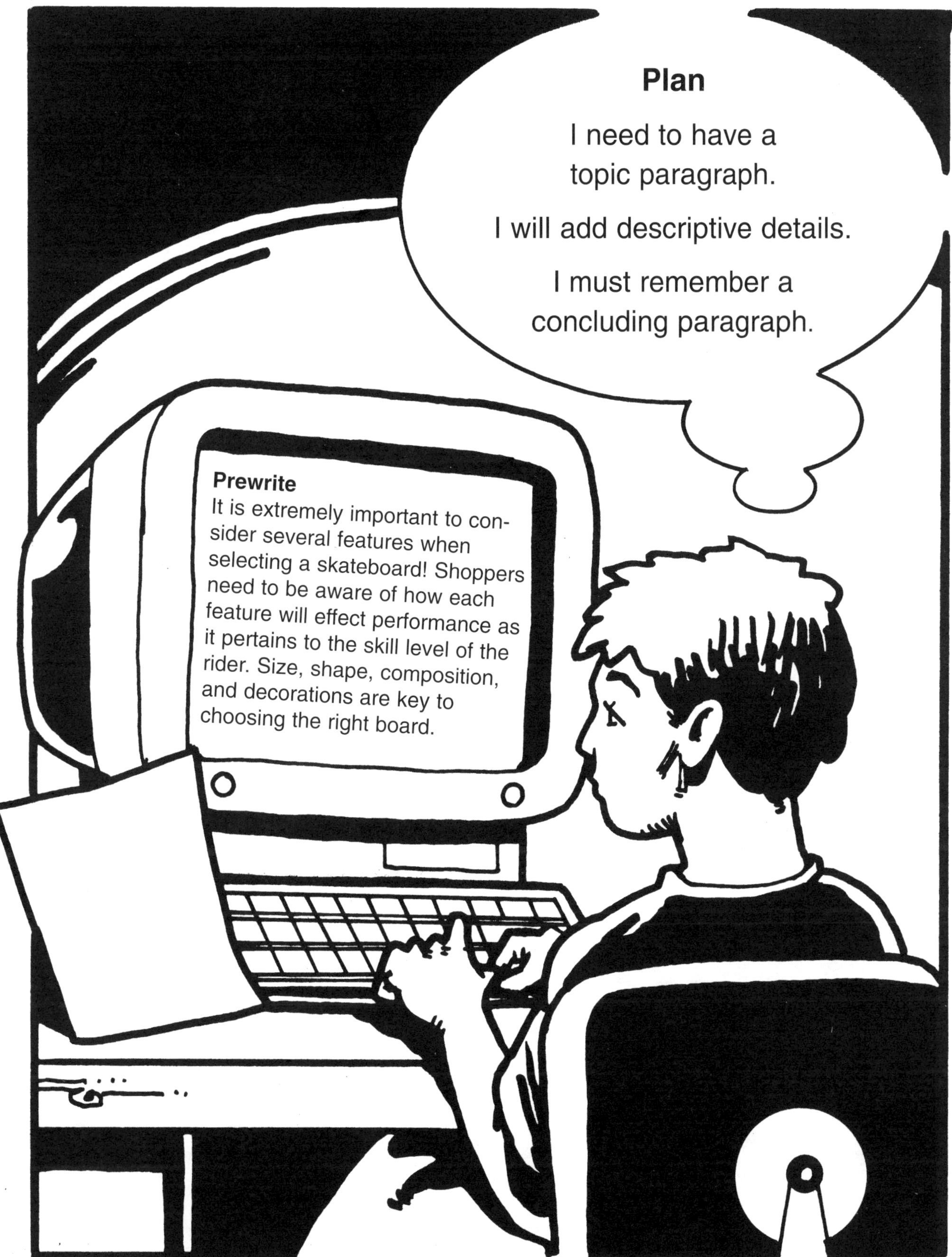

© 2001 *Thinking Publications.* Duplication permitted for educational use only.

Rapid Write

CODE-SWITCHING TOOLS ONE

Date: ______________________________

Name: ____

Directions

- My job is to code switch 4 sentences.
- I'll need this paper and a pencil.
- I'll know I'm finished when I have rewritten 4 complete sentences using correct punctuation.
- When I'm finished I'll share this work with the teacher.

Rewrite these sentences using a different code.

1. Today was a real bummer at school. I'm ready to go home and chill out!

____

____

2. My new video game has radical graphics. It's awesome!

____

____

3. I blew off studying for my math test and bombed it!

____

____

4. Sam's got a really cool bike! He catches major air off the ramp.

____

____

© 2001 *Thinking Publications.* Duplication permitted for educational use only.

CODE-SWITCHING TOOLS: IDENTIFYING SUBJECTS AND VERBS

GOAL

To recognize and use subjects and verbs

BACKGROUND INFORMATION

In the previous lesson *(Code-Switching Tools: Introducing Communication Registers),* students learned the concept of changing communication registers to accomplish a variety of communication tasks, which strengthened their metalinguistic skills, such as flexible use of vocabulary in oral and written language. The purpose of this lesson is to provide students with an opportunity to identify and use different parts of speech as tools for switching communication registers and expanding spoken and written language. Specifically, this lesson will target identification of subjects and verbs in sentences. The next two lessons will focus on adverbs / adjectives and synonyms.

OBJECTIVES

1. Identify and use the following vocabulary: *subject, verb,* and *noun.*
2. Identify subjects and verbs in sentences.
3. Use a graphic code to mark subjects and verbs in sentences.

MATERIALS

1. *Use Word Power to Code Switch!* poster (Created earlier)
2. *Code-Switching Tools* graphic (See page 98; duplicate and enlarge the graphic, color it, mount it onto construction paper or poster board, and laminate it for durability if desired.)
3. *Baby Whale's Journey* (1999) by Jonathan London (This book was selected because of its high interest level, descriptive language, interesting subject matter, and simple sentence structure. Any book with similar characteristics can be substituted.)
4. *Rapid Write: Code-Switching Tools Two* (See page 99; duplicate one per student.)

INTRODUCTION

Tie-in to Prior Learning

Remind students that in the last lesson they accepted a "mission possible" and learned about using word power to code switch between three styles of language. Ask students if they remember the three language codes. Elicit the terms *social language, work/school/community language,* and *written language.*

Tell students that they will be concentrating on the words used to switch codes in this lesson and the next two lessons.

Focus/Relevance

Refer to the *Use Word Power to Code Switch!* poster. Explain that a secret agent might use special tools (e.g., a shoe with a telephone built into the heel or a camera built into a pen) to complete a mission. Tell students that they will also be learning about some special tools to help them make the switch to the communication codes they will need for school, work, or community success. Show the *Code-Switching Tools* poster. Tell students that their special tools will be lines and shapes around words in sentences that will tell them the types of words they are reading. Point to the lines under subject and verb. Explain that the code-cracking job in this lesson will be to identify the subject and verb of sentences with these special tools.

LESSON ACTIVITIES

1. Show the cover of *Baby Whale's Journey.* Ask students what they know about whales. Elicit information about a whale's size, habitat, or endangered species status. Ask students the following questions: "Did you know that sperm whales need air to breathe but can hold their breath for more than an hour when diving for food? Did you know that they rest vertically and lie motionless when sleeping?" Explain that students will be using ideas from this interesting book to practice two of the tools on the *Code-Switching Tools* poster.

2. Write the following sentence where everyone can see it:

   Whales rest vertically.

   Ask students which part of the sentence is the subject. Point out that they might have talked about parts of a sentence in language arts classes during previous grades. Using the *Code-Switching Tools* poster, review the criteria for the subject of a sentence (i.e., the subject tells what or who is doing the action and is usually a noun, pronoun, or noun phrase). Using the whale sentence, explain that you will identify the subject by underlining it. Underline the word *whales.*

3. Ask students which part of the sentence is the verb. Using the *Code-Switching Tools* poster, review the criteria for a verb in a sentence (i.e., the verb tells the action). Again, using the sentence, model a code for identifying the verb by drawing a zigzag line under the word *rest.*

4. Read "Facts about Sperm Whales" from the Readers Guide section on the last page of the book (or read a similar section). Have students practice identifying the subject and verb of

the sentences. Explain that as the story is read, they will be identifying subjects and verbs of longer, more complicated sentences. Read *Baby Whale's Journey* to students and stop occasionally to have students identify the subjects and verbs in sentences. Explain that to switch a code, sometimes you just need to choose a different subject or verb.

5. Hand out *Rapid Write: Code-Switching Tools Two*. Read through the directions as a group and check for understanding. Explain to students that their job is to use codes to mark the subjects and verbs in each sentence. Remind students to underline the subjects and put a zigzag line under the verbs. Remind students to reread for clarity before asking for help or finishing their work. Check responses as a group.

CLOSURE

Summarize the lesson, review its relevance to students, and tie it to future learning. Explain that in the next lesson *(Code-Switching Tools: Elaborating with Adverbs and Adjectives)* they will be identifying more tools to help code switch.

Code-Switching Tools

Subject Tells what or who.

The baby whale swam.

Verb Tells the action.

The duck followed its mother.

Adverb Describes a verb by telling…

How *(quickly)* When *(today)*
Where *(outside)* Degree *(barely)*

Adjective Describes a noun.

The giant squid attacked.

Synonym Means the same as or is similar to another word.

big = giant, enormous, huge

© 2001 *Thinking Publications.* Duplication permitted for educational use only.

Rapid Write

CODE-SWITCHING TOOLS TWO

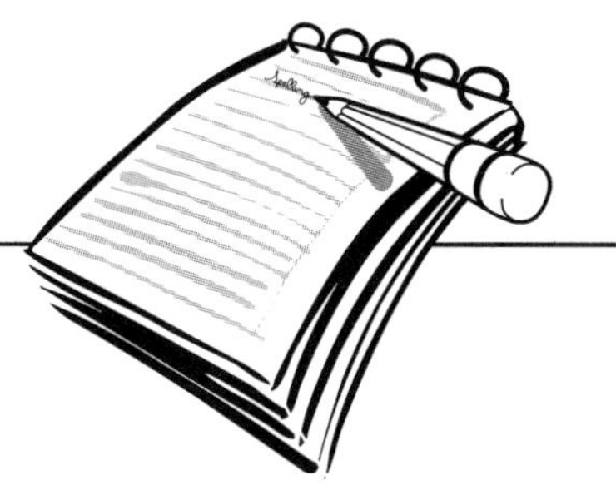

Date: ____________________________

Name: ____

Directions

- My job is to mark the subject with an underline and the verb with a zigzag line in each sentence.
- I'll need this paper and a pencil.
- I'll know I'm finished when every sentence has 2 "codes."
- When I'm finished I'll share this work with the teacher.

Mark the subject with an underline and the verb with a zigzag line.

1. Whales breathe air.
2. Whales communicate.
3. Sea animals swim gracefully.
4. The ocean is salty.
5. Giant squids attack whales.
6. Two whales circle each other.
7. The mother whale nudges the baby to the surface.
8. The mother whale spots a shark as it approaches her baby.
9. The mother whale has won.
10. Baby whale feasts.

© 2001 *Thinking Publications.* Duplication permitted for educational use only.

CODE-SWITCHING TOOLS: ELABORATING WITH ADVERBS AND ADJECTIVES

GOAL

To recognize and use adverbs and adjectives

BACKGROUND INFORMATION

In the previous lessons *(Code-Switching Tools: Introducing Communication Registers* and *Code-Switching Tools: Identifying Subjects and Verbs),* students learned the three communication registers (i.e., social language, work/school/community language, and written language) and practiced identifying subjects and verbs. The purpose of this lesson is to provide students with an opportunity to identify and use other parts of speech as tools for switching communication registers and expand their spoken and written language. Specifically, this lesson will focus on the use of adverbs and adjectives as tools for elaborating sentences.

OBJECTIVES

1. Identify and use the terms *adverb* and *adjective.*
2. Identify adverbs and adjectives within sentences.
3. Use a graphic code to mark adverbs and adjectives in sentences.
4. Expand simple sentences by adding adverbs and adjectives.

MATERIALS

1. *Code-Switching Tools* poster (Created earlier)
2. *Endangered Species Sentences* (see page 103; duplicate one per student.)
3. *Rapid Write: Code-Switching Tools Three* (See page 104; duplicate one per student.)

INTRODUCTION

Tie-in to Prior Learning

Remind students that in the last lesson they identified subjects and verbs in sentences. Ask students if they remember the codes they used when identifying subjects and verbs. The subject was usually the noun, pronoun, or noun phrase that performed the action while the verb was usually the word or words that completed the action. Review using this sentence: *The baby whale swam close to its mother.* Have students identify the subject and verb.

Focus/Relevance

Tell students that in this lesson they will learn to use more code-switching tools to build word power. Ask students if they have ever heard the terms *adverb* or *adjective* in their language arts classes. Explain that these are two important parts of speech that can be used when code switching. Remind students that using more powerful words to code switch can help them "win" at school with better grades, "win" in the job market by being able to find good jobs, and "win" with their friends because they will be more powerful communicators.

LESSON ACTIVITIES

1. Refer to the *Code-Switching Tools* poster, and highlight the shapes associated with adverbs (triangles) and adjectives (rectangles). Draw a large triangle and a large rectangle where everyone can see them. Explain that an adverb describes how, when, where, or the degree to which the action is performed and an adjective describes a noun. Write this sentence near the shapes:

   The student carefully packed his torn backpack.

2. Have one student identify the verb in the sentence by drawing a zigzag line under the word *packed*. Draw a large triangle around the word *carefully*. Ask a student to pantomime the action described in the sentence. Discuss situations that might cause a student to perform this action *carefully* (e.g., trying to keep the torn backpack together or packing something fragile). Change the word in the triangle to *quickly* and ask a different student to pantomime the new sentence meaning. Once again, discuss situations that would cause the difference in the action. Emphasize that in this sentence, the adverb describes or modifies the verb by telling *how* it is performed (e.g., carefully or quickly). Choose volunteers to demonstrate the following situations, and let the other students brainstorm adverbs that could be added to describe how the action was performed.

   Situations:

   - I walked home from the field after loosing the big game.
   - The shy student asked the teacher for a pencil.
   - I told the dog not to chew on my shoes.
   - The scientist mixed the chemicals.
   - The hungry students lined up for lunch.
   - The silly clown removed her makeup.
   - The wild horse bucked the rider off.
   - The frozen milk shake melted in the hot sun.

Possible adverb choices:

suddenly	quietly	gently
quickly	calmly	cautiously
politely	happily	slowly
carelessly	nervously	proudly
cheerfully	impatiently	angrily

Point out the large triangle drawn earlier, and write the word *adverb* in the triangle. Explain that this is the code for identifying adverbs.

3. Point out the large rectangle drawn earlier, and write the word *adjective* in the rectangle. Remind students that an adjective describes a noun. Highlight the word *backpack* in the example sentence and draw a large rectangle around the word *torn.* Tell students that adjectives are wonderful tools for describing the five senses (i.e., how something looks, feels, sounds, tastes, or smells). List other words under the rectangle that they could use to describe a backpack (e.g., large, blue, or leather).

4. Hand out *Endangered Species Sentences.* Model the directions by underlining the subject, drawing a zigzag line under the verb, and drawing shapes over the adverbs and adjectives as a group activity. Guide students in coding the parts of speech for the remaining sentences. Discuss their responses. Explain that adverbs and adjectives can be added to sentences or changed in sentences when code switching.

   NOTE: To make this activity even more visual and hands-on, create an overhead of *Endangered Species Sentences* and use transparent colored geometric shapes to identify the parts of speech.

5. Hand out *Rapid Write: Code-Switching Tools Three*. Read through the directions as a group and check for understanding. Ask students to use the *Code-Switching Tools* poster to fill in the sentences with the appropriate type of word. Remind students to reread for clarity before asking for help or finishing their work. Discuss their responses.

CLOSURE

Summarize the lesson, review its relevance to students, and tie it to future learning. Compliment students on their use of codes to identify subjects, verbs, adverbs, and adjectives. Tell students that in the next lesson *(Code-Switching Tools: Elaborating with Synonyms)* they will practice using synonyms to expand their code-switching tools.

Endangered Species Sentences

Name: ______________________________ Date: ____________________

Underline the subject in each sentence. Draw a zigzag line under the verb. Draw a triangle around the adverb and a rectangle around the adjective.

1. The cunning tiger runs silently and swiftly.
2. The blue whale gently caresses her baby.
3. The huge Indian elephant sprays water everywhere with its long trunk.
4. Lazily, the old crocodile sleeps in the sun.
5. The snow leopard crouches silently on a high branch.
6. A graceful, strong bald eagle circles slowly overhead.
7. A three-toed sloth carefully hangs from a branch.
8. Patiently, the male penguin holds his precious eggs on his feet throughout the entire winter.
9. Giant pandas eagerly eat large amounts of bamboo plants every year.
10. Arctic seals carelessly frolic and splash in the icy ocean.

© 2001 *Thinking Publications.* Duplication permitted for educational use only.

Rapid Write

CODE-SWITCHING TOOLS THREE

Date: ______________________

Name: ____________________________________

Directions

- My job is to add adverbs and adjectives to 5 sentences.
- I'll need this paper and a pencil.
- I'll know I'm finished when I have added 5 adverbs in the triangles and 5 adjectives in the rectangles.
- When I'm finished I'll share this work with the teacher.

Add an adverb to each triangle and an adjective to each rectangle.

1. The [ ] explorer clung △ to the steep mountainside.
2. The [ ] bald eagle swooped △ into the water to catch a fish.
3. △, the experienced sailor tied a knot in the [ ] rope to secure the sails.
4. Indians and colonists △ approached one another to trade [ ] furs for metal tools.
5. The raccoon △ snuck into the camp and feasted on a variety of [ ] foods.

© 2001 *Thinking Publications.* Duplication permitted for educational use only.

CODE-SWITCHING TOOLS: ELABORATING WITH SYNONYMS

GOAL

To recognize and use synonyms

BACKGROUND INFORMATION

Previously in this unit, students learned the three communication registers and practiced identifying subjects, verbs, adverbs, and adjectives in sentences. The purpose of this lesson is to provide students with an opportunity to identify and use a variety of interesting vocabulary words (i.e., synonyms) to expand and elaborate their spoken and written language. This lesson completes the code-switching tools lessons.

OBJECTIVES

1. Understand and use the term *synonym.*
2. Generate synonyms for given words or phrases.
3. Refine and edit sentences using synonymous word choices.

MATERIALS

1. Travel magazine (e.g., *National Geographic)*
2. *My Artic Visit* (See page 108; duplicate one per student.)
3. Previously created Unit Two posters *(Use Word Power to Code Switch!* and *Code-Switching Tools)*
4. *Toad* (1999) by Ruth Brown (This book was chosen because of its repeated pattern of listing synonyms and its relationship to the curriculum. Any book with similar characteristics can be substituted.)
5. *Rapid Write: Code-Switching Tools Four* (See page 109; duplicate one per student.)
6. *Just Do It! Review Activity Two* (See page 110; duplicate one per student.)

INTRODUCTION

Tie-in to Prior Learning

Remind students that in the last lesson *(Code-Switching Tools: Elaborating with Adverbs and Adjectives)* they added to their code-switching tools by identifying and using adverbs and adjectives in sentences. Write a boring sentence where everyone can see it (e.g., *The dog slept under the tree*). Have students identify the subject and the verb of the sentence and share ideas for improving the sentence by adding adjectives and adverbs (e.g., *The small dog slept lazily under the green shady tree*). Applaud their creativity. Explain that in this lesson students will learn a way to make their word choices even more *compelling*—purposely use this complex word at this point in the lesson without explaining its meaning.

Focus/Relevance

1. Bring in a travel magazine (e.g., *National Geographic*) to set the stage. Tell students to pretend that they are editors for a major travel magazine. Hand out *My Arctic Visit* and read it together. Ask students to pretend that they are the editor who wrote this paragraph, and ask for their opinions regarding the intentionally dull and repetitive text. Elicit the idea that the paragraph uses the same words over and over rather than using a variety of words that have more word power. After determining that the paragraph needs refining before it is ready for publication, tell students that they will be improving the paragraph by using a variety of word choices, or *synonyms*, for the verbs and adjectives.

2. Explain that rather than working on this paragraph right away, students will return to it once they have had some practice identifying synonyms from a story about creature from a vastly different habitat. Elicit some guesses as to what might be a stark contrast to an arctic environment (e.g., a swamp).

LESSON ACTIVITIES

1. Refer to the *Code-Switching Tools* poster, and highlight the oval shape associated with synonyms. Ask students if they have heard the word *synonym* in other classes. Have one student explain the word *synonym*. Then say the following two sentences: "The sand is hot. The sand is burning." Emphasize that the meaning of the sentences stayed the same while the word choice changed. Ask students to name the book that is a fabulous source of synonyms (i.e., a thesaurus). Point out that some word-processing programs for computers include a thesaurus. Challenge students to take advantage of this tool when writing.

2. Show students the book *Toad*. Tell them that the author of the book makes a big impact by including synonyms to make her writing more interesting. Show the cover of *Toad* and ask students to describe it. Make predictions about the content of the book based on the cover. Discuss the setting. Start reading the story. Stop after a few pages, and ask students what they notice about the words in the sentences (i.e., the frequent use of adjectives). Highlight synonymous word pairs that are interesting as the book is read, including:

   foul, filthy; lumps, bumps; stains, spots; septic, toxic; clumsy, careless; sticky, gooey

   Discuss how much more interesting language becomes when synonyms are used.

3. As a group activity, use a thesaurus to edit *My Arctic Visit*. Guide students in identifying and circling boring words. Tell students that although a thesaurus is a great tool when writing for almost any purpose, their brain can be an equally powerful tool for generating synonyms. Tell students that they are going to test this theory by playing "Brains versus Book." To play, one student (i.e., the Book) looks up a word (e.g., *cold)* in the thesaurus while other students (i.e., the Brains) brainstorm synonyms for the word. The Book does not share any of his or her findings until the Brains have generated a list. After the Brains complete their list, the list is compared to the number of words found in the thesaurus by the Book. Emphasize that students' brains can be just as effective as a thesaurus!

4. Using the list, edit *My Arctic Visit* as a group. Allow students to take turns choosing interesting synonyms. Reread the paragraph with the synonyms added. Tell students that they now have a compelling article for publication. Ask students why the term *compelling* is a good description of their work. Elicit or offer the synonyms *interesting, exciting, attention grabbing,* and *thrilling.* Briefly discuss the importance of synonyms to a travel magazine editor (e.g., synonyms help to attract travelers to the location or subscribers to the magazine) and to students when they code switch.

5. Hand out *Rapid Write: Code-Switching Tools Four*. Read through the directions as a group and check for understanding. Stress that the use of a thesaurus is optional for this assignment. Have students work independently on editing the sentences. Remind students to reread for clarity before asking for help or finishing their work. Discuss their responses.

CLOSURE

Summarize the lesson, review its relevance to students, and tie it to future learning. Comment on how students have used careful and powerful word choices when elaborating with synonyms. Have students give examples of when this skill would be useful to them. Explain that in the next lesson *(Word Power: Comparing and Contrasting)* they will learn more about word power by comparing and contrasting.

JUST DO IT!

Hand out *Just Do It! Review Activity Two.* Explain that this is a homework activity that reviews the code-switching lessons from Unit Two. Refer to the previously created Unit Two posters *(Use Word Power to Code Switch!* and *Code-Switching Tools).* Briefly review vocabulary from the posters. Review the directions for *Just Do It! Review Activity Two.* Set a due date for the assignment.

My Artic Visit

I visited an arctic habitat and it was very cold!

The cold wind went down my collar.

Snow was everywhere!

Penguins stood together to keep warm and protect their eggs from the cold weather.

My nose was as cold as an ice cube!

Polar bears fished in the cold Arctic Ocean water.

If you visit the arctic habitat, be sure to bring your thermal underwear because it's so cold there!

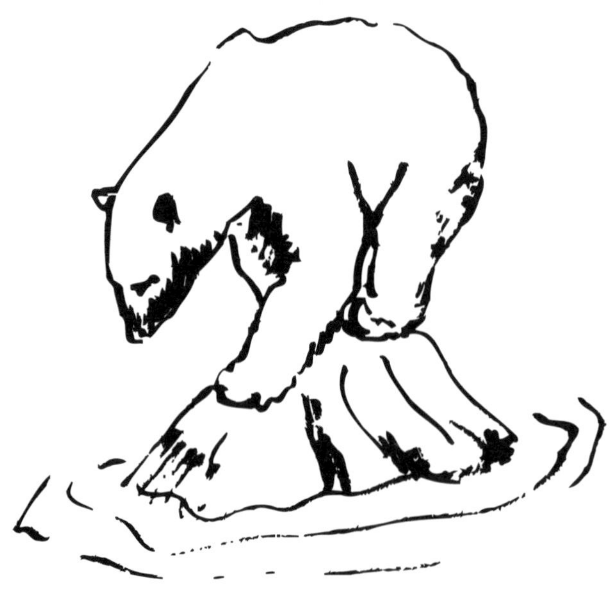

© 2001 *Thinking Publications.* Duplication permitted for educational use only.

RAPID WRITE

CODE-SWITCHING TOOLS FOUR

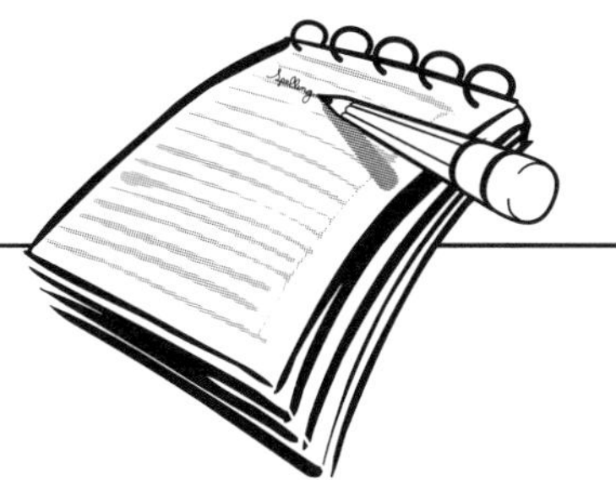

Date: ___________________________

Name: ____

Directions

- My job is to improve the 4 items using synonyms.
- I'll need this paper, a pencil, and a thesaurus (if desired).
- I'll know I'm finished when I have crossed out 8 words and have written 8 synonyms above the words.
- When I'm finished I'll share this work with the teacher.

Cross out the boring words that are in bold print and write a more powerful synonym in the space above each sentence.

complex ecosystem

Example: The pond habitat is a ~~**busy place**~~ where many creatures find food and make their home.

1. Ducks walk along the muddy lakeshore looking for **good** materials, such as twigs and moss, to build a nest. Beavers walk along the creek looking for sticks to build a **good** dam.

2. Frogs **catch** flies with their sticky tongues while spiders **catch** mosquitoes in their webs.

3. Fish **eat** insects and bits of plants floating in the water. Green herons, which are large birds, **eat** fish that swim to the surface to catch bugs.

4. All the organisms depend on the pond environment in **many** different ways. From the small insects to the thirsty deer, **many** creatures require the pond community for survival.

© 2001 *Thinking Publications.* Duplication permitted for educational use only.

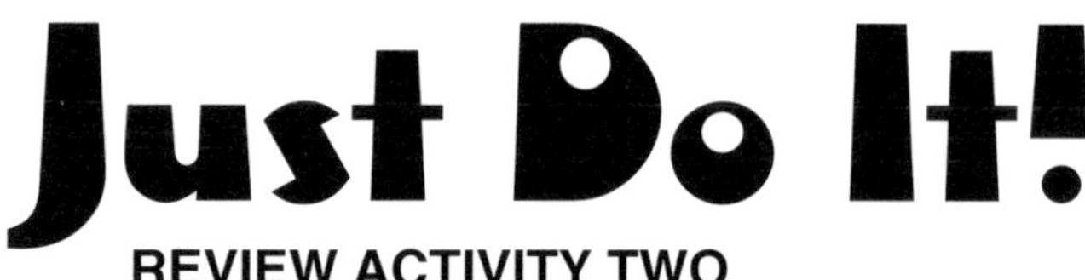

REVIEW ACTIVITY TWO

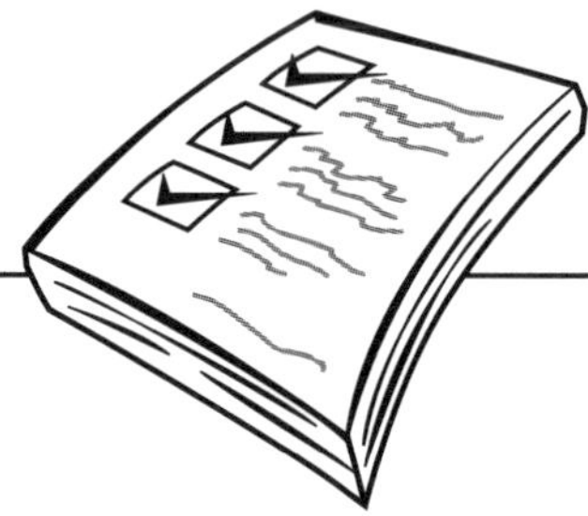

Complete the following tasks with a family member.
Initial each after you've completed it.

_____ Explain *code switching.* What changes could you make when switching from social language to work/school/community language and written language?

_____ Greet someone using social language.

_____ Greet someone using work/school/community language.

_____ Describe how you could say hello using written language (e.g., when writing a letter).

_____ Tell the codes you would use to identify the *subject,* the *verb,* the *adverb,* and the *adjective* in this sentence:

Busy students worked happily.

_____ Give an adverb, an adjective, and a synonym to elaborate the following sentences:

- My **puppy** was happy. (adjective)
- He **jumped** up and down. (adverb)
- We went for a **walk.** (synonym)

Student signature: ______________________________

Family member signature: ______________________________

This review activity is due back at school on:

© 2001 *Thinking Publications.* Duplication permitted for educational use only.

WORD POWER: COMPARING AND CONTRASTING

GOAL

To compare and contrast items

BACKGROUND INFORMATION

The purpose of this lesson is to provide students with a strategy for comparing and contrasting concepts both orally and in writing. Students will identify similarities and differences between two items and develop a strategy for using spoken and written language to convey that information. This lesson strengthens metalinguistic skills, such as flexible use of vocabulary in both oral and written language activities.

OBJECTIVES

1. Understand and use the terms *compare* and *contrast.*
2. Use a graphic organizer to compare and contrast concepts and terms.
3. Compare and contrast items in a short written exercise.

MATERIALS

1. *Use Word Power to Code Switch!* poster (Created earlier)
2. *Use Word Power to Compare and Contrast!* graphic (See page 114; duplicate and enlarge the graphic, color it, mount it onto construction paper or poster board, and laminate it for durability if desired; also duplicate one copy per student.)
3. *Turn of the Century* (1998) by Ellen Jackson (This book was chosen because it provides historical information from the perspective of children living at 100-year intervals from the year 1000 to the year 2000. The clever combination of fiction and factual information engages children and adults. The book provides excellent opportunities for comparing and contrasting; it also directly supports classroom curriculum concepts. Any book with similar characteristics can be substituted.)
4. *Rapid Write: Word Power* (See page 115; duplicate one per student.)

INTRODUCTION

Tie-in to Prior Learning

Ask students to summarize the strategy for improving their word power that they learned for code switching. Refer to the *Use Word Power to Code Switch!* poster. Remind students that they learned to make better word choices by using synonyms in the last lesson *(Code-Switching Tools: Elaborating with Synonyms)*. Tell students that this lesson will teach them another tool for increasing their word power.

Focus/Relevance

Discuss the special event that happened on January 1, 2001 (i.e., the end of one century and the start of another). Ask students if they think they could have anything in common with a child who lived 100 years ago. Have students predict what they think the life of a child was like back then. Ideas for comparison include conveniences, transportation, and play-time activities. Ask the same question about children who lived 1,000 years ago. Tell students that they might be surprised to know that though their lives would be very different there are many ways in which they would be alike.

LESSON ACTIVITIES

1. Show the *Use Word Power to Compare and Contrast!* poster. Discuss the terms *compare* and *contrast.* Explain that *compare* means to look for similarities and *contrast* means to look for differences. Explain the Venn diagram on the poster. When two items are compared to each other, the overlapping parts of the circle hold similarities about the two items and the outside parts of each circle list differences. Demonstrate the use of the strategy by having students think of three similarities between a clock and a calendar. Highlight that they both track the passing of time, they both have numbers, and they both can be hung on a wall. Tell students that these three similarities would be listed in the overlapping section of the circles. Next, have students brainstorm how a calendar and a clock are different from one another. Highlight that a clock and a calendar are different: a clock tracks time in minutes and hours, has twelve daytime and twelve nighttime hours, and has a face and hands; a calendar tracks time over days and months, is usually made from paper, and lists the twelve months of the year. Tell students that the differences are listed on either side of the similarities, within the nonoverlapping sections of the circles. Tell students that knowing how to compare and contrast can help them in their classes. The graphic organizer can help them organize ideas when speaking or writing.

2. Show the cover of the book *Turn of the Century*. Ask students what they notice about the illustrations on the cover. Elicit the idea of seeing both old-fashioned and modern buildings and vehicles. Explain that this book is exciting because it gives interesting details about the lives of boys and girls who lived long ago. Read through the first few pages, and then select highlights from subsequent pages. Choose a time period from the book that connects to a curriculum concept (e.g., if students are studying a colonial unit, the page describing the 1800s might be an appropriate selection).

3. Refer to the *Use Word Power to Compare and Contrast!* poster while you draw a Venn diagram where everyone can see it. Select two time periods from the book to compare and contrast. As students brainstorm ideas, use bullet points and make brief notes. After the group discusses the similarities and differences, have one student summarize the ideas orally using complete sentences.
4. Hand out *Rapid Write: Word Power* and a copy of the *Use Word Power to Compare and Contrast!* poster. Read through the directions as a group and check for understanding. Review the *Use Word Power to Compare and Contrast!* poster and use of the Venn diagram as a prewriting organizer. Have students choose two things to compare and contrast. Ask students to write three similarities for the three items chosen and two differences for each item on their copy of *Use Word Power to Compare and Contrast!* Then summarize their ideas on *Rapid Write: Word Power.* Remind students to reread for clarity before asking for help or finishing their work. Have students share their responses.

CLOSURE

Summarize the lesson, review its relevance to students, and tie it to future learning. Compliment students on their use of a comparing and contrasting strategy to organize their thoughts and use specific vocabulary to compare and contrast. Ask students when this would be an important skill (e.g., when organizing a writing assignment, when making decisions, or when shopping). Explain that they have already laid the foundation for the next strategy by looking for similarities or patterns. Ask students if they enjoy working with puzzles or solving mysteries. The next lesson *(Discover the Pattern: Solving Analogy Relationships)* will involve thinking about puzzles called *analogy patterns.*

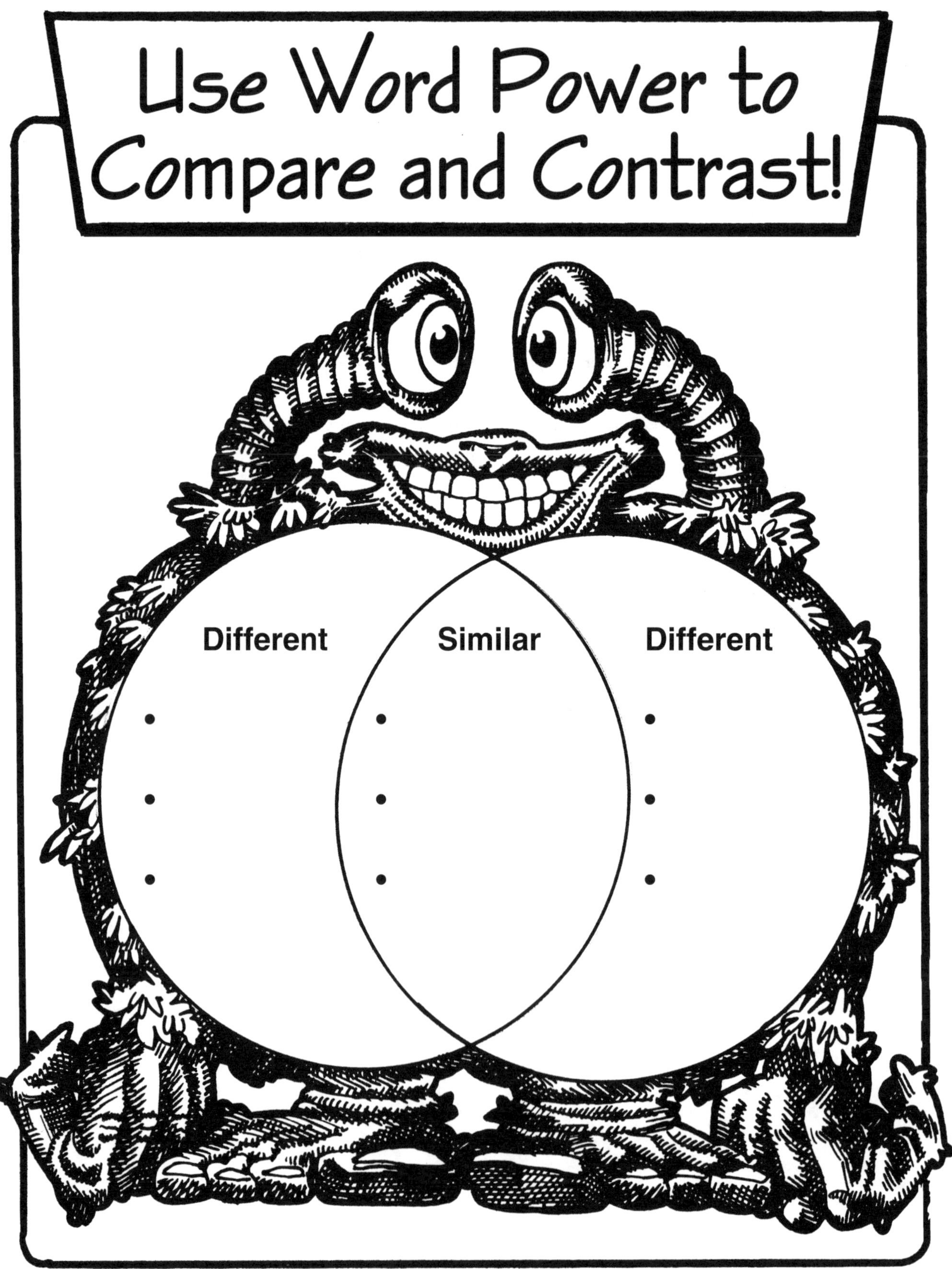

© 2001 *Thinking Publications.* Duplication permitted for educational use only.

RAPID WRITE

WORD POWER

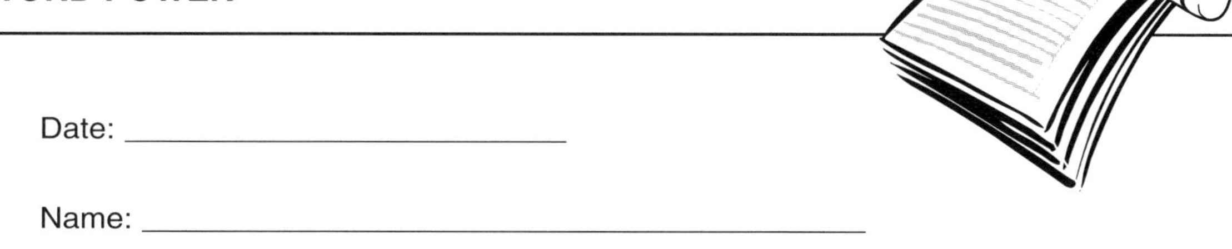

Date: ____________________

Name: ______________________________

Directions

- My job is to use a graphic organizer to compare and contrast 2 things.
- I'll need this paper, the *Use Word Power to Compare and Contrast!* poster, and a pencil.
- I'll know I'm finished when I have written 6 differences and 3 similarities in the graphic organizer and written 6 complete sentences on this page.
- When I'm finished I'll share this work with the teacher.

Choose 2 things to compare and contrast. Organize your ideas with the *Use Word Power to Compare and Contrast!* poster. Then put your ideas into complete sentences.

Compare and contrast

____________________ **and** ____________________

1. Similarities

•

•

•

2. Differences

•

•

•

© 2001 *Thinking Publications.* Duplication permitted for educational use only.

DISCOVER THE PATTERN: SOLVING ANALOGY RELATIONSHIPS

GOAL

To recognize relationships between words

BACKGROUND INFORMATION

The purpose of this lesson is to apply word power strategies to solving analogy patterns. Solving analogies requires students to recognize word relationships and describe the relationship using higher level vocabulary. As in the previous lessons in Unit Two, this lesson also strengthens metalinguistic skills, such as flexible use of vocabulary in both oral and written language activities.

OBJECTIVES

1. Recognize relationships between words.
2. Understand and use the following terms: *antonym, synonym, member-category, location, function, characteristic,* and *part-whole.*
3. Complete analogy patterns.

MATERIALS

1. *Discover the Pattern* graphic (See page 118; duplicate and enlarge the graphic, color it, mount it onto construction paper or poster board, and laminate it for durability if desired.)
2. *Analogy Pattern Cards* (See pages 119–126; duplicate the cards, laminate for durability if desired, and cut apart.)
3. *Rapid Write: Discover the Pattern* (See page 127; duplicate one per student.)

INTRODUCTION

Tie-in to Prior Learning

Remind students that in the last lesson *(Word Power: Comparing and Contrasting)* they practiced comparing and contrasting children who lived during different centuries. Explain that in this lesson they will practice comparing and contrasting word meanings to solve analogy patterns. Discuss the concept of a pattern (i.e., information that is repeated in a predictable sequence). Have students brainstorm examples of patterns.

Focus/Relevance

Show the *Discover the Pattern* poster, and point out that an analogy is a comparison between two things that are similar in some way. To discover an analogy pattern, students must first figure out what the relationship is between the first two words in the puzzle and then create a similar relationship for the next two words. Review the poster and model how the symbols ":" and "::" are read. Tell students that ":"means "is to" and "::" means "as" or "in the same way as." Have students give examples of each relationship on the *Discover the Pattern* poster and use the appropriate terms when stating the relationship aloud. Review the analogy relationships: antonym, synonym, member-category, location, function, characteristic, and part-whole. Tell students that these are all possible relationships between words that can form a pattern. Knowing these patterns can help students link new words to words they already know, allowing them to remember new words. Read the analogy example from the poster (i.e., entrance : exit :: rough : _________) and discuss possible answers. Remind students they must identify the pattern at the beginning of the analogy before they can fill in a pair of words that will match the pattern.

LESSON ACTIVITIES

1. Show the stack of *Analogy Pattern Cards,* and explain that each of the cards has an analogy pattern on it that will match one of the relationships on the *Discover the Pattern* poster. Shuffle the cards and deal them to students. Have students volunteer to read a card, identify the relationship from the *Discover the Pattern* poster, and complete the analogy. As an option, students could write the analogy responses on a blank card or a piece of paper.

   NOTE: There are nine cards for each relationship in the set of *Analogy Pattern Cards.*

2. Once a student has completed the analogy, have other students look at their cards to see if their word pairs have a similar relationship. Continue until all the analogies have been solved. Students can also create their own analogies. Notice that there is one blank card provided that may be duplicated so students can create analogies for others to solve.

3. Hand out *Rapid Write: Discover the Pattern.* Read through the directions as a group and check for understanding. Ask students to make up seven words pairs to demonstrate each relationship. Remind students to reread for clarity before asking for help or finishing their work. Discuss their responses.

CLOSURE

Summarize the lesson, review its relevance to students, and tie it to future learning. Remind students that if they can recognize the pattern they can solve the analogy. Knowing how words are related will help them remember new words. Tell students that they will continue to use their word power to define words in the next lesson *(Smooth Sailing: Giving Clear Definitions).*

Discover the Pattern

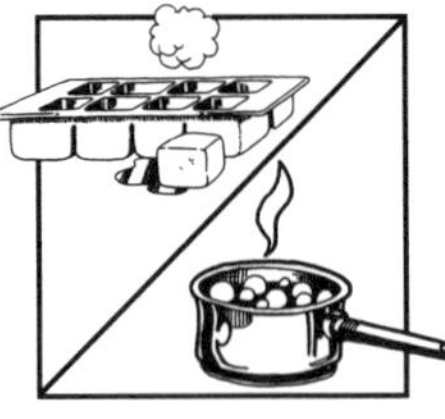

Antonym
cold : hot

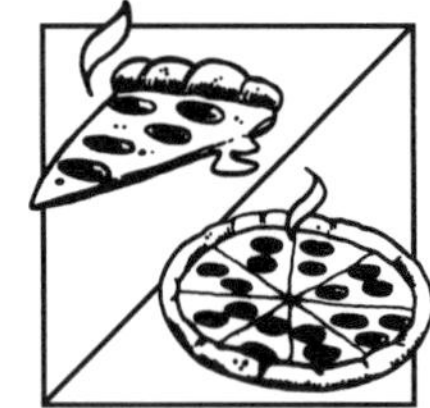

Part-Whole
slice : pizza

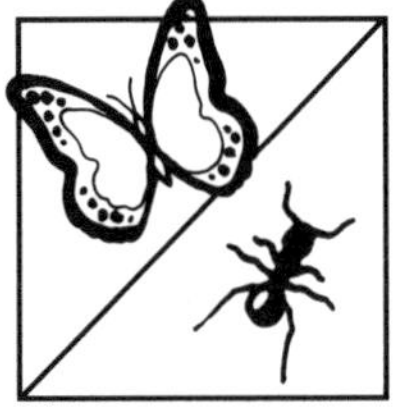

Synonym
insect : bug

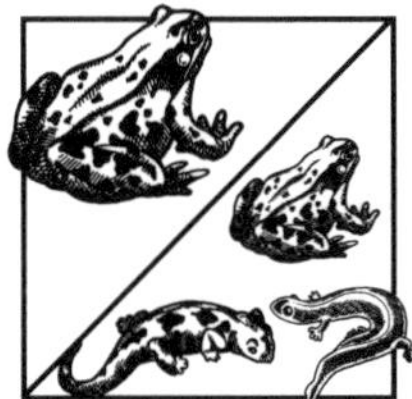

Member-Category
frog : amphibian

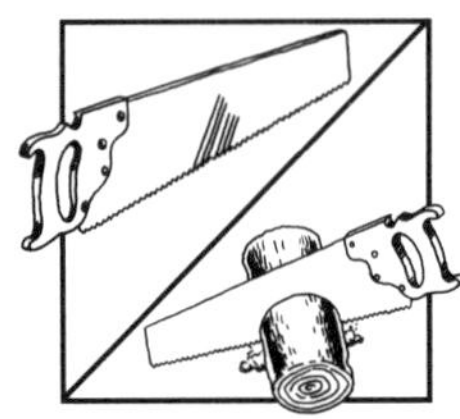

Function
saw : cut

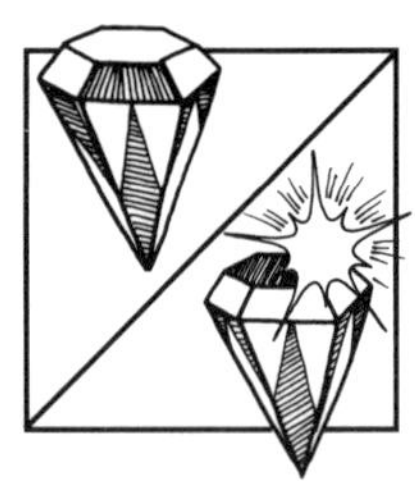

Characteristic
diamond : shiny

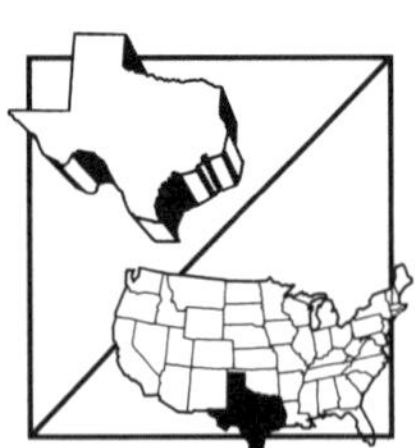

Location
state : country

entrance : exit :: rough : ________

© 2001 *Thinking Publications.* Duplication permitted for educational use only.

Analogy Pattern Cards

terrific : marvelous :: ________ : ________	old : ancient :: ________ : ________
recall : remember :: ________ : ________	gift : present :: ________ : ________
buy : purchase :: ________ : ________	insect : bug :: ________ : ________
look : gaze :: ________ : ________	bashful : shy :: ________ : ________

© 2001 *Thinking Publications.* Duplication permitted for educational use only.

brave : courageous

::

_______ : _______

lead : follow

::

_______ : _______

near : far

::

_______ : _______

borrow : lend

::

_______ : _______

against : for

::

_______ : _______

fancy : plain

::

_______ : _______

entrance : exit

::

_______ : _______

increase : decrease

::

_______ : _______

© 2001 *Thinking Publications.* Duplication permitted for educational use only.

rough : smooth

::

__________ : __________

shark : ocean

::

__________ : __________

lower : raise

::

__________ : __________

skier : slope

::

__________ : __________

baby : crib

::

__________ : __________

bracelet : wrist

::

__________ : __________

waiter : restaurant

::

__________ : __________

doctor : hospital

::

__________ : __________

© 2001 *Thinking Publications.* Duplication permitted for educational use only.

owl : forest

::

_______ : _______

bones : body

::

_______ : _______

planets : space

::

_______ : _______

wings : airplane

::

_______ : _______

cactus : desert

::

_______ : _______

skin : snake

::

_______ : _______

hands : clock

::

_______ : _______

doorknob : door

::

_______ : _______

© 2001 *Thinking Publications.* Duplication permitted for educational use only.

whiskers : cat
::
________ : ________

hearts : beat
::
________ : ________

stars : flag
::
________ : ________

fingers : grasp
::
________ : ________

bark : tree
::
________ : ________

bee : pollinate
::
________ : ________

cornea : eye
::
________ : ________

map : guide
::
________ : ________

© 2001 *Thinking Publications.* Duplication permitted for educational use only.

whistle : blow :: ________ : ________	clown : funny :: ________ : ________
ruler : measure :: ________ : ________	sweater : warm :: ________ : ________
oven : heat :: ________ : ________	firefighter : courageous :: ________ : ________
fan : cool :: ________ : ________	judge : fair :: ________ : ________

© 2001 *Thinking Publications.* Duplication permitted for educational use only.

broom : sweep

::

_____ : _____

mathematics : school subjects

::

_____ : _____

monkey : noisy

::

_____ : _____

pants : clothing

::

_____ : _____

rainbow : colorful

::

_____ : _____

soccer : sports

::

_____ : _____

orange : juicy

::

_____ : _____

Memorial Day : holidays

::

_____ : _____

© 2001 *Thinking Publications.* Duplication permitted for educational use only.

bowling ball : heavy

::

__________ : __________

bus : transportation

::

__________ : __________

popcorn : salty

::

__________ : __________

cake : desserts

::

__________ : __________

bed : furniture

::

__________ : __________

engineer : occupation

::

__________ : __________

poodle : dogs

::

__________ : __________

__________ : __________

::

__________ : __________

© 2001 *Thinking Publications.* Duplication permitted for educational use only.

Rapid Write

DISCOVER THE PATTERN

Date: ______________________________

Name: ____

Directions

- My job is to write an example of each relationship in the spaces.
- I'll need this paper and a pencil.
- I'll know I'm finished when I have 7 word pairs.
- When I'm finished I'll share this work with the teacher.

Write an example of each relationship.

1. Antonym ________________ : ________________
2. Synonym ________________ : ________________
3. Member-Category ________________ : ________________
4. Location ________________ : ________________
5. Function ________________ : ________________
6. Characteristic ________________ : ________________
7. Part-Whole ________________ : ________________

© 2001 *Thinking Publications.* Duplication permitted for educational use only.

SMOOTH SAILING: GIVING CLEAR DEFINITIONS

GOAL

To define words

BACKGROUND INFORMATION

The purpose of this lesson is to help students become aware of what makes a clear and precise definition and to use this information when defining words orally and in writing. This lesson relies on students' knowledge of strategies that have been taught in the previous two lessons. Students are taught that a clear definition includes a consideration of how the word is used (i.e., the part of speech), describes the category the word belongs in, describes the word's distinctive features, and (if appropriate) gives a specific example. As in previous lessons in Unit Two, this lesson strengthens metalinguistic skills, such as flexible use of vocabulary in both oral and written language activities.

OBJECTIVES

1. Use context clues to learn the meaning of a word.
2. Define words using precise vocabulary.

MATERIALS

1. Previously created Unit Two posters (*Use Word Power to Compare and Contrast!* and *Discover the Pattern)*
2. *The Mary Celeste: An Unsolved Mystery from History* (1999) by Jane Yolen and Heidi Elisabet Yolen Stemple (This book was chosen for its definitions that provide factual information about ships and its nautical information from the 1800s. The mysterious nature of the story is highly motivating for students, and the historical information lends itself to curriculum concepts of exploration, transportation, immigration, and history. Any book with similar characteristics can be substituted.)
3. *Smooth Sailing with Clear Definitions* graphic (See page 132; duplicate and enlarge the graphic, color it, mount it onto construction paper or poster board, and laminate it for durability if desired.)
4. *Rapid Write: Smooth Sailing* (See page 133; duplicate one per student.)
5. *Just Do It! Review Activity Three* (See page 134; duplicate one per student.)

INTRODUCTION

Tie-in to Prior Learning

Remind students that in the last lesson *(Discover the Pattern: Solving Analogy Relationships)* they practiced solving analogy patterns. Refer students back to the *Use Word Power to Compare and Contrast!* poster and the *Discover the Pattern* poster and review the word power concepts on the posters. Explain that in this lesson students will continue to develop their word power as they tell and write definitions.

Focus/Relevance

Ask students what the word *mystery* means. Elicit the idea of trying to figure out who or what did something. Ask how mysteries are usually solved. Elicit the idea of looking for clues, gathering evidence, and forming a hypothesis or educated guess about the event. Show the cover of the book *The Mary Celeste*. Ask students what they think the mystery might be. Tell students that this book is about a real event that happened over 130 years ago and that no one has been able to figure it out. They will be using their word power to figure out many of the words in the book. Ask what the word *nautical* means. Discuss that for the moment the word *nautical* might be a mystery but by the end of this lesson they will have the tools to solve this mystery.

LESSON ACTIVITIES

1. Ask students what they do when they come across a word that they do not know. Discuss the different strategies students might use (e.g., using context clues, looking in a dictionary or glossary, or skipping over the word and continuing to read). Write the word *bow* where everyone can see it, and without reading the word aloud, ask students what this word means. Discuss ideas presented by students (e.g., a decoration for your hair or for a package, the action of bending downward or lowering the head to greet or show respect, a weapon for shooting arrows, or a tool for playing a stringed instrument). Discuss the importance of knowing the context of how a word is used before being able to tell the meaning. Stress that the context will tell how the word is used (e.g., as a noun, a verb, an adjective, or an adverb). Ask what the meaning of the word is based on the context clues from the following sentence:

   As we reached the United States, I stood on the bow of the ship, so I could be the first to spot the Statue of Liberty.

   Ask a student to look up the word *bow* in the dictionary and read the various definitions. Have students listen and signal when they hear the appropriate definition read.

2. Show the *Smooth Sailing with Clear Definitions* poster, and review each part of a clear definition. Point out that a clear definition should include the following:

- A grammatical use (the part of speech the word represents)
- A category (the larger group the word belongs to)
- A distinctive feature (what makes it special; its function, composition)
- A specific example (if appropriate)

Offer the following as examples:

Ship (noun)—*It's a kind of transportation, a large seagoing vessel* (e.g., The Titanic is a famous ship).

Ship (verb)—*The* action of *sending or transporting something from one place to another* (e.g., I shipped the package on Saturday).

NOTE: Encourage students to avoid using the word being defined (e.g., run = To run fast) though it is acceptable to use the defined word in an example. Also tell students that when writing a definition, they might use the word to start the sentence (e.g., A ship is…).

3. Explain that having a strategy for being able to explain word meanings using a clear definition is important at school, at home, and in the community. It is important for students to be clear whenever they need to explain a term or concept to others.

4. Begin reading the story. Stop to highlight vocabulary and define words using the poster as a guide. Lead students through the first few words, allowing them to become more independent as the story progresses. Tell students that they will use sentences from *The Mary Celeste* to write clear definitions. Highlight the following literary component:

   - Vocabulary—*mystery, danger, journey, navigation, theory, hypothesis, ocean, whale, state, wave, stern, flag, hail, log, register, hold, oar, mutiny, berth, cargo, salvage, run*

5. Hand out *Rapid Write: Smooth Sailing*. Read through the directions as a group and check for understanding. Ask students to write complete definitions for the three underlined words from the story *The Mary Celeste.* Remind students to reread for clarity before asking for help or finishing their work. Let students share their written sentences as time allows.

CLOSURE

Summarize the lesson, review its relevance to students, and tie it to future learning. Let students share their hypotheses of the ill-fated vessel. Refer back to the *Smooth Sailing with Clear Definitions* poster, stressing the important components of a clear definition. Ask a student to give a definition for *The Mary Celeste.* Challenge students to apply this strategy in all of their classes, at home, and in the community.

JUST DO IT!

Hand out *Just Do It! Review Activity Three.* Explain that this is a homework activity covering the strategies they have learned so far in the last three lessons. Refer to the previously created posters from Unit Two. Briefly review concepts from the posters. Review the directions for *Just Do It! Review Activity Three.* Set a due date for the assignment.

Smooth Sailing with Clear Definitions

- **How is the word used?**
  (Noun, verb, adverb, adjective)

- **What category is it in?**

- **What are its distinctive features?**
  (Function, composition, location, appearance)

- **Are there any specific examples?**

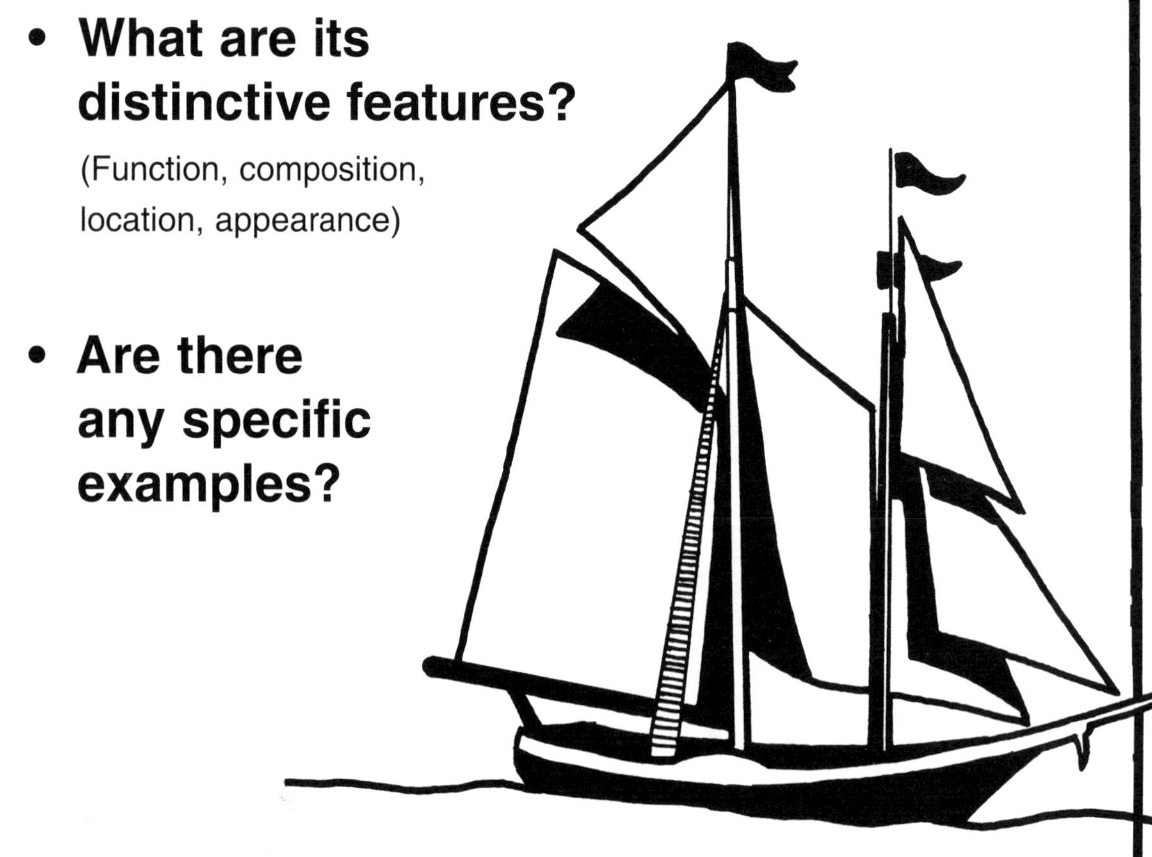

© 2001 *Thinking Publications.* Duplication permitted for educational use only.

Rapid Write

SMOOTH SAILING

Date: ____________________

Name: ______________________________

Directions

- My job is to write 3 definitions in complete sentences with correct punctuation.
- I'll need this paper and a pencil.
- I'll know I'm finished when I have written 3 definitions that include the part of speech, the category the word belongs to, distinctive features, and a specific example (if appropriate).
- When I'm finished I'll share this work with the teacher.

Write a definition for each underlined word in the following sentences.

1. The log from an enormous tree was cut into lumber for building a ship called *The Mary Celeste.*

____

____

2. I can see the flag wave when the wind blows.

____

____

3. The state of Texas is one of the largest in the country.

____

____

© 2001 *Thinking Publications.* Duplication permitted for educational use only.

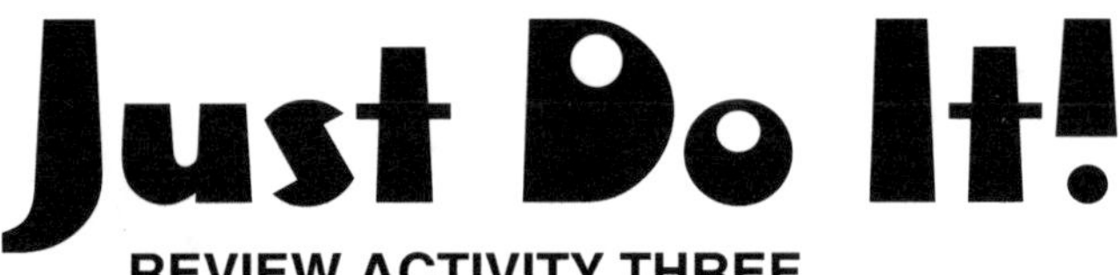

REVIEW ACTIVITY THREE

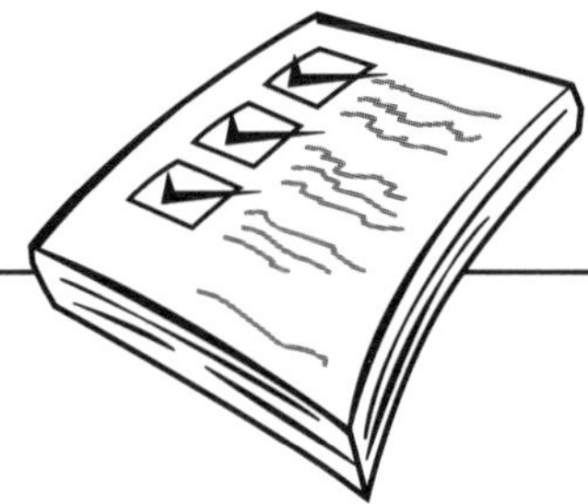

Complete the following tasks with a family member. Initial each after you've completed it.

____ Use a graphic organizer to compare and contrast pizza and hamburgers. Then summarize your thoughts for a family member.

____ Make up 7 word pairs using each analogy relationship once. Use objects around your home. Analogy relationships: *antonym, synonym, member-category, location, function, characteristic,* and *part-whole.*

____ Give a clear definition for the word *state* by telling its grammatical use, the category, distinctive features, and a specific example (if applicable).

- State (noun)
- State (verb)

Examples:

Ship (noun)—*It's a kind of transportation, a large seagoing vessel* (e.g., The Titanic is a famous ship).

Ship (verb)—*The action of sending or transporting something from one place to another* (e.g., I shipped the package on Saturday).

This review activity is due back at school on:

Student signature ______________________________

Family member signature ______________________________

© 2001 *Thinking Publications.* Duplication permitted for educational use only.

ULTIMATE WORD POWER TOOLS: USING SIMILES AND METAPHORS

GOAL

To understand and use figurative language

BACKGROUND INFORMATION

The purpose of this lesson is to begin to expose students to figurative language that will help them more creatively express a thought or feeling. Specifically, students will learn about similes and metaphors. Similes and metaphors make comparisons that create mental images for the listener or reader. The comparison is meant to bring spoken and written language to life.

In the next lesson *(Extreme Communication: Using Figurative Language)*, figurative language will be further explored with idiomatic expressions, puns, and jokes. Students will learn the role figurative language plays in humor and social communication. As in previous lessons in Unit Two, this lesson strengthens metalinguistic skills, such as flexible use of vocabulary in both oral and written language activities.

OBJECTIVES

1. Identify similes and metaphors in speaking and writing.
2. Express a thought or feeling using a simile or metaphor.
3. Use similes and metaphors in a structured writing activity.

MATERIALS

1. *Smooth Sailing with Clear Definitions* poster (Created earlier)
2. Sports picture (Cut from a magazine or newspaper.)
3. *Figurative Language: Taking Communication to the Extreme!* graphic (See page 138; duplicate and enlarge the graphic, color it, mount it onto construction paper or poster board, and laminate it for durability if desired.)
4. Poetry selections (Find selections that use humor or whimsy or that employ the beauty of descriptive, figurative language. Whimsical or humorous examples may be found in poetry, such as *Where the Sidewalk Ends* [1974] by Shel Silverstein.)
5. *Rapid Write: Ultimate Word Power Tools* (See page 139; duplicate one per student.)

INTRODUCTION

Tie-in to Prior Learning

Remind students that in the last lesson *(Smooth Sailing: Giving Clear Definitions)* they worked on telling and writing clear definitions to explain word meanings. Review the information that must be included in a definition by referring to the *Smooth Sailing with Clear Definitions* poster. Tell students that in this lesson they will be using what they know about clear definitions to build vivid word pictures in the minds of their listeners and readers.

Focus/Relevance

Show a picture of a person participating in a sport (e.g., an Olympic gymnast leaping through the air), and ask students to brainstorm sentences to describe what they see. Let several students make up descriptive sentences and write them where everyone can see them. Compliment students on their use of word power strategies. Tell students that in this lesson they will be adding a new, extremely powerful tool to their collection of word power strategies: figurative language.

LESSON ACTIVITIES

1. Show the *Figurative Language: Taking Communication to the Extreme!* poster and read the simile and metaphor examples. Highlight the terms *simile* and *metaphor.* Tell students that they can use these ultimate word power tools to make understanding what they hear easier and make writing more powerful. Explain that by using figurative language they will be using many of the strategies they learned in previous Unit Two lessons. Have students generate other examples of similes and metaphors orally in class for extra practice.

2. Use the sentence from the Focus/Relevance section, and have students highlight the subject of the sentence by underlining it. Have them identify the verb, adjectives, and adverbs and code them as was done in earlier lessons. Let students brainstorm synonyms to replace words and then read the new and improved sentences.

   Next, tell students that words can also be added to create a simile or a metaphor. Similes and metaphors compare the athlete to something else. For example, a graceful gymnast could be compared to other graceful things to paint a vivid picture. Have students brainstorm a list of things that are graceful. Refer to the *Figurative Language: Taking Communication to the Extreme!* poster, and point out the comparisons made for the snowboarder and surfer. Choose a word from the lists to illustrate the two forms of figurative language. Highlight the following rules:

- Simile—Uses *like* or *as.*
  The gymnast *was as graceful as a gazelle* leaping through the air.
- Metaphor—Uses a form of "be" (e.g., is, are, was, were)
  The gymnast *was a gazelle* leaping through the air.

Write the following sentences where everyone can see them, and as a group code and edit them by adding a simile or metaphor. Show students how to identify keywords to help them write the simile or metaphor.

- *The hockey puck slid quickly across the ice.*
- *The basketball player's feet banged loudly as he raced across the floor.*
- *The skater spun in a tight circle on the sparkling ice.*

3. Tell students that authors and poets often use similes and metaphors in their work because it can help readers picture the idea in their head. Read a selected poem that uses figurative language. Identify and discuss the similes and metaphors used by the author. Share and discuss a selected poem that uses humorous or whimsical language.
4. Hand out *Rapid Write: Ultimate Word Power Tools*. Read through the directions as a group and check for understanding. Remind students to identify the key subjects, verbs, adjectives, and adverbs and then brainstorm metaphors or similes to fit. Remind students to reread for clarity before asking for help or finishing their work. Let students share their responses as time allows.

CLOSURE

Summarize the lesson, review its relevance to students, and tie it to future learning. Congratulate students on their use of ultimate word power tools to describe things in a completely different way! Tell students that in the next lesson *(Extreme Communication: Using Figurative Language)* they will be taking the use of figurative language to the extreme!

Figurative Language
Taking Communication to the Extreme!
Idiom
Mountain climbers
"take their life into their hands"
when scaling a cliff.
Use the
Ultimate
Word Power
Tools!
Simile
The snowboarder slid
like a snake down
the mountain.
Metaphor
The surfboard was a
torpedo speeding
across the water.

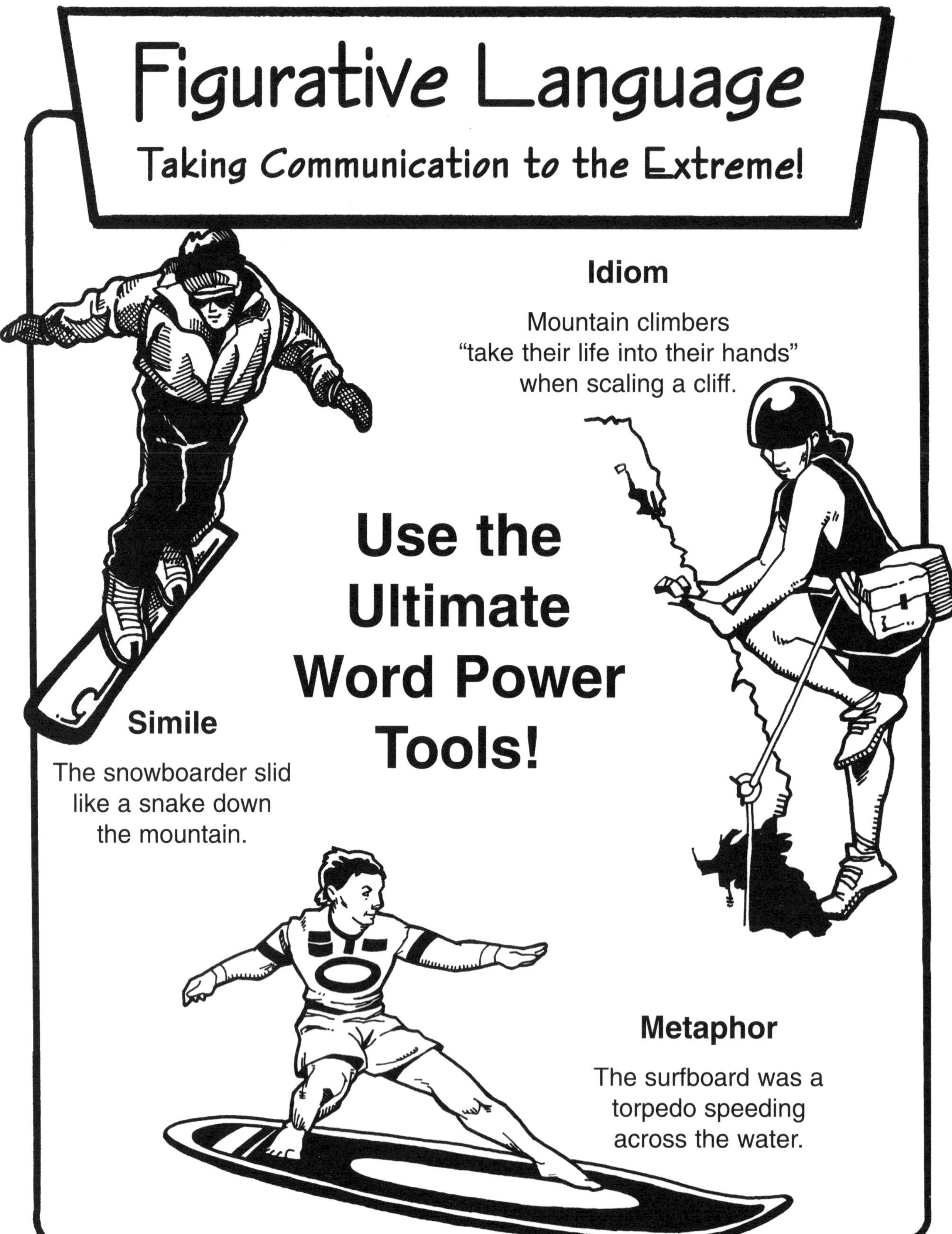

© 2001 *Thinking Publications.* Duplication permitted for educational use only.

Rapid Write

ULTIMATE WORD POWER TOOLS

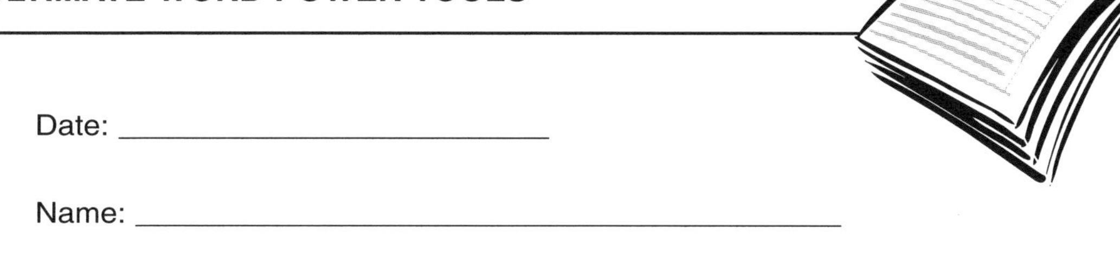

Date: ______________________

Name: ______________________________________

Directions

- My job is to write similes or metaphors to complete the sentences.
- I'll need this paper and a pencil.
- I'll know I'm finished when I have filled in 10 sentences.
- When I'm finished I'll share this work with the teacher.

Circle the keywords that will help you complete each simile or metaphor. Then write a word or phrase that completes each metaphor or simile.

Examples: The kayak (bobbed) through the rapids like a cork.
The bicycle was a rocket (speeding) down the steep hill.

1. The quarterback's pass was like ______________________ as it sailed to the end zone.
2. The motocross racer was ______________________ shooting through the air.
3. The trophy was as shiny as ______________________.
4. The ball was ____________ soaring above the catcher's mitt.
5. The skaters were as fast as ________________ as they raced to the finish line.
6. The gymnast was like ________________ as she flipped through the air.
7. The snowbank is ____________ waiting to trap a skier.
8. The blades on the ice skates were as sharp as ____________.
9. The fans, in their bright colors, looked like ________________ cheering in the stands.
10. The crack of the bat sounded like ________ in the quiet stadium.

© 2001 *Thinking Publications.* Duplication permitted for educational use only.

EXTREME COMMUNICATION: USING FIGURATIVE LANGUAGE

GOAL

To understand and use figurative language

BACKGROUND INFORMATION

In the previous lesson *(Ultimate Word Power Tools: Using Similes and Metaphors)*, similes and metaphors were used to creatively express a thought or feeling. In this lesson, the knowledge of figurative language is extended. The purpose of this lesson is to expose students to a variety of figurative language forms including multiple meaning words, puns, jokes, and idiomatic expressions. Briefly expose students to the different figurative language uses or expand the activities for an in-depth application.

OBJECTIVES

1. Recognize the literal and figurative meanings of idiomatic expressions and multiple meaning words in a variety of figurative language uses (i.e., puns, jokes, idioms, metaphors, and similes).
2. Use the knowledge of figurative and literal meanings of idiomatic expressions in a structured writing activity.

MATERIALS

1. *Figurative Language: Taking Communication to the Extreme!* poster (Created earlier)
2. Any joke, riddle, or poetry book that provides examples of a variety of figurative language forms (e.g., *See the Yak Yak* [1999] by Charles Ghigna and *Tough Cookie* [1999] by David Wisniewski)
3. *Rapid Write: Extreme Communication* (See page 143; duplicate one per student.)
4. *Just Do It! Review Activity Four* (See page 144; duplicate one per student.)

INTRODUCTION

Tie-in to Prior Learning

Remind students that in the last lesson *(Ultimate Word Power Tools: Using Similes and Metaphors)* they learned two forms of figurative language. Ask students to name the tool that compares two things using *like* or *as* (e.g., I felt as hot as a burning log in a fireplace). Elicit the term *simile.* Then ask for the name of the tool that compares two things using a form of *be* (e.g., The sun is a fiery furnace in space). Elicit the term *metaphor.* Refer back to the *Figurative Language: Taking Communication to the Extreme!* poster.

Focus/Relevance

Tell students that this lesson is called *Extreme Communication.* Ask a student to define the word *extreme.* Elicit the concepts of "pushing the envelope," "reaching the greatest point or degree," and "the max." Explain that in this lesson they will need all of their word power tools to tackle an extreme communication challenge.

LESSON ACTIVITIES

1. Without telling students what the extreme communication challenge is, read the following:
   - *The hockey puck missed the goal "by a mile."*
   - *I've got "cold feet" about giving my speech.*
2. Have students explain one of the jokes. Point out the play on words involved in the jokes. Tell students that just as similes and metaphors can be used to create a vivid picture in a listener's or reader's mind, idioms and multiple meaning word plays called *puns* also create powerful and humorous pictures in our minds. However, emphasize that when listening to a joke that uses humor based on figurative language, students might be confused if they picture the literal meaning in order to "get it." If students picture the literal meaning, they have misunderstood and may be confused. Ask students if they have ever heard anyone tell a joke that they did not understand.
3. Write the words *literal* and *figurative* where everyone can see them. Using the "cold feet" joke, draw the literal meaning next to the word *literal.* Remind students to use the context clues and figure out the part of speech that is being used. If students picture the figurative meaning of "cold feet" (i.e., being scared or nervous), congratulate them for getting the joke.
4. Discuss that in everyday language, figurative expressions are not always used for humor. When we picture the ideas in our heads exactly as the words are said, we may be thinking of the *literal* meaning of the expression. If this happens, it will not make sense and won't fit the situation. Ask a student to illustrate by drawing a picture of the literal meaning for the phrase, "When you turned in your terrific science project it *knocked my socks off!"* Discuss the context clues from the sentence, and ask students to tell the real message of *knocked my socks off.* Next to the word *figurative,* write the real message (i.e., the teacher was pleased or excited).
5. Read more jokes from a variety of sources to allow students an opportunity to understand various figurative language expressions.

6. Hand out *Rapid Write: Extreme Communication.* Read through the directions as a group and check for understanding. Allow students time to independently complete the activity. Remind students to reread for clarity before asking for help or finishing their work. Allow time for students to share their work.

CLOSURE

Summarize the lesson, review its relevance to students, and tie it to future learning. Congratulate students on completing Unit Two! Encourage them to listen carefully at school, at home, and in the community for the context clues that signal a figurative expression, so they do not miss the boat! Explain that in the next unit (Unit 3) they will begin to use all their word power to get a handle on telling stories.

JUST DO IT!

Hand out *Just Do It! Review Activity Four.* Explain that this is a homework activity covering the last two lessons. Refer to the *Figurative Language: Taking Communication to the Extreme!* poster. Briefly review vocabulary from the poster. Review the directions for *Just Do It! Review Activity Four.* Set a due date for the assignment.

Rapid Write

EXTREME COMMUNICATION

Date: ____________________________

Name: ____

Directions

- My job is to draw the literal meaning for an idiom and then write a sentence to explain the real meaning of the idiom.
- I'll need this paper and a pencil.
- I'll know I'm finished when I have drawn the literal meaning of the expression and written a sentence explaining what the expression really means.
- When I'm finished I'll share this work with the teacher.

Analyze the meaning of this idiom:

Let's put our heads together and solve this problem!

Draw the literal meaning (the cartoon would look like…).

Write the figurative meaning (this expression really means…).

____

____

© 2001 *Thinking Publications.* Duplication permitted for educational use only.

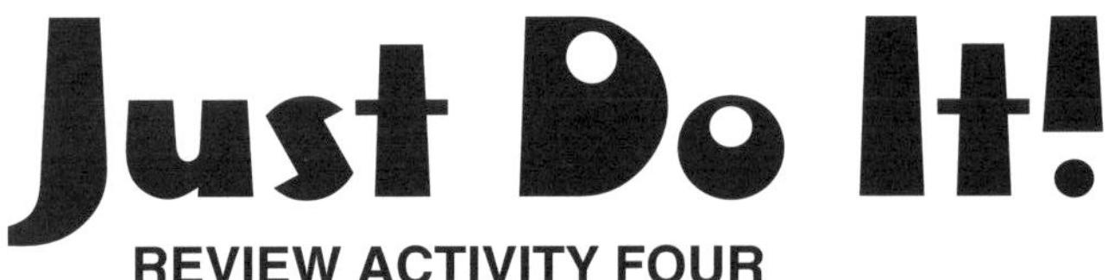

REVIEW ACTIVITY FOUR

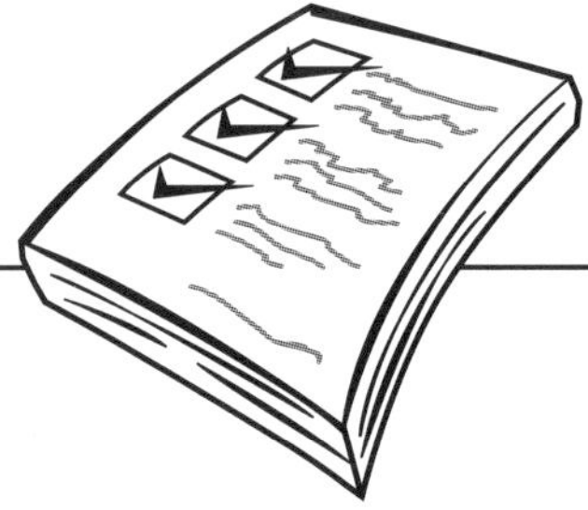

Complete the following tasks with a family member.
Initial each after you've completed it/

___ Use context clues to tell a word or phrase to complete the similes or metaphors.

- My bike was a ____ flying down the hill.
- I was as free as a _______________________ after I finished my homework and chores.
- The water slide is like a ____.
- The basketball was a _________________________ swooshing into the bucket.

___ Explain the figurative meaning of the expressions in quotations.

- I could have raked leaves for extra money, but I slept late and "missed the boat."
- I "hit it on the head" when I answered the question.
- I "nailed it" on the first try!
- I have my "work cut out for me."

This review activity is due back at school on:

Student signature _______________________________________

Family member signature __________________________________

© 2001 *Thinking Publications.* Duplication permitted for educational use only.

UNIT THREE

GOAL-SETTING ACTIVITY THREE

GOAL

To encourage self-improvement through goal setting

BACKGROUND INFORMATION

The purpose of this lesson is to help students learn the steps for setting and meeting a goal (i.e., identifying a need, formulating a goal, practicing the steps to reach the goal, revising the goal as needed, and evaluating progress) and apply the steps to setting a goal for working with stories. Rather than expecting students to set goals independently, the goal-setting process is modeled. Writing a story knowledge goal could be teacher directed, but reflection on the need for the goal and how the goal might be useful will be individual for each student since each student's use of the goal is different.

OBJECTIVES

1. Evaluate progress on achieving the previous goal.
2. Tell how the previous goal was met.
3. Write a goal related to knowledge of story structure.

MATERIALS

1. Unit Two posters
2. *Goal Setting: Activity Two* (Each student's previously completed goal sheet.)
3. *Goal Setting: Activity Three* (See page 150; duplicate one per student.)

INTRODUCTION

Tie-in to Prior Learning

Compliment students on their hard work during the Unit Two to improve their word power skills at school, both orally and in writing. Remind students that in *Goal-Setting Activity Two* they identified specific word power skills that could be focused on for improvement. Refer to posters from Unit Two, and use them for discussion while completing activities in this lesson.

Focus/Relevance

1. Write the word *evaluate* where everyone can see it. Review the concept of using evaluation as a tool to decide whether students have successfully completed their goal.

2. Remind students that learning is easier when goals are set and there is a plan for practicing. Setting goals can help students achieve many different skills in school, at home, and someday at work. Discuss how it feels to accomplish something that was difficult. Then tell students that it is time to evaluate their progress on the goals set in Unit Two.

LESSON ACTIVITIES

1. Hand out each student's copy of *Goal Setting: Activity Two.* Refer to each of the Unit Two posters. Encourage students to reflect on the steps they took to achieve the goal written on their goal sheet as well as how the goal has been helpful at home, in school, or in the community. Remind students that they will want to continue to practice each completed goal while targeting a new one.

2. Give each student a copy of *Goal Setting: Activity Three.* Remind students that in the previous unit they practiced an important part of communication by learning to use word power strategies in many different situations. Explain to students that in this unit they will be learning about the parts of a story, so they can become better listeners/readers and storytellers/authors. Expand on this concept by discussing a story and deciding what makes a logical and clear story. Elicit ideas, such as beginning, middle, end, climax, good language, main ideas, and details.

3. Write the words *story knowledge* where everyone can see them, and tell students that they will have an important goal to achieve for this unit. Write the following goal where everyone can see it:

   I will recognize story elements and use them to tell or write better stories.

4. Read through *Goal Setting: Activity Three* as a group and check for understanding. Have students complete the goal statements on their goal sheets by adding the word *elements.* Tell students to write down examples of situations when story knowledge may be used at home, at school, or in the community. Remind students to reread for clarity before asking for help or finishing their work. Discuss their responses.

   HINT: If students have difficulty generating situations, use one of the following ideas:

   An example of when this goal is important

   - at home is when I have to tell my mother why something happened.
   - at school is when I have to describe how the civil war started.
   - in the community is when I tell my friend about a good movie I just saw.

CLOSURE

Summarize the lesson, review its relevance to students, and tie it to future learning. Recap for students by explaining that they have set an important goal and in the next lesson they will begin working on the first step to achieve their goal. Have them sign and date *Goal Setting: Activity Three.* By signing and dating the goal sheet, they are promising to concentrate and work on the goal. Explain that you will also sign the goal sheets as a promise to help each student reach his or her goal. Encourage students to take the goal sheet home to share with their family, but request that they must return it by a set time with a family member's initials. Keep the goal sheets for future reference as they will be handed out and reviewed at the end of the unit. When the goal sheets are returned, you might want to keep them all in one folder or create a separate folder for each student.

HINT: Offer a tangible or social reward for returning the goal sheet with a family member's initials.

GOAL SETTING

ACTIVITY THREE

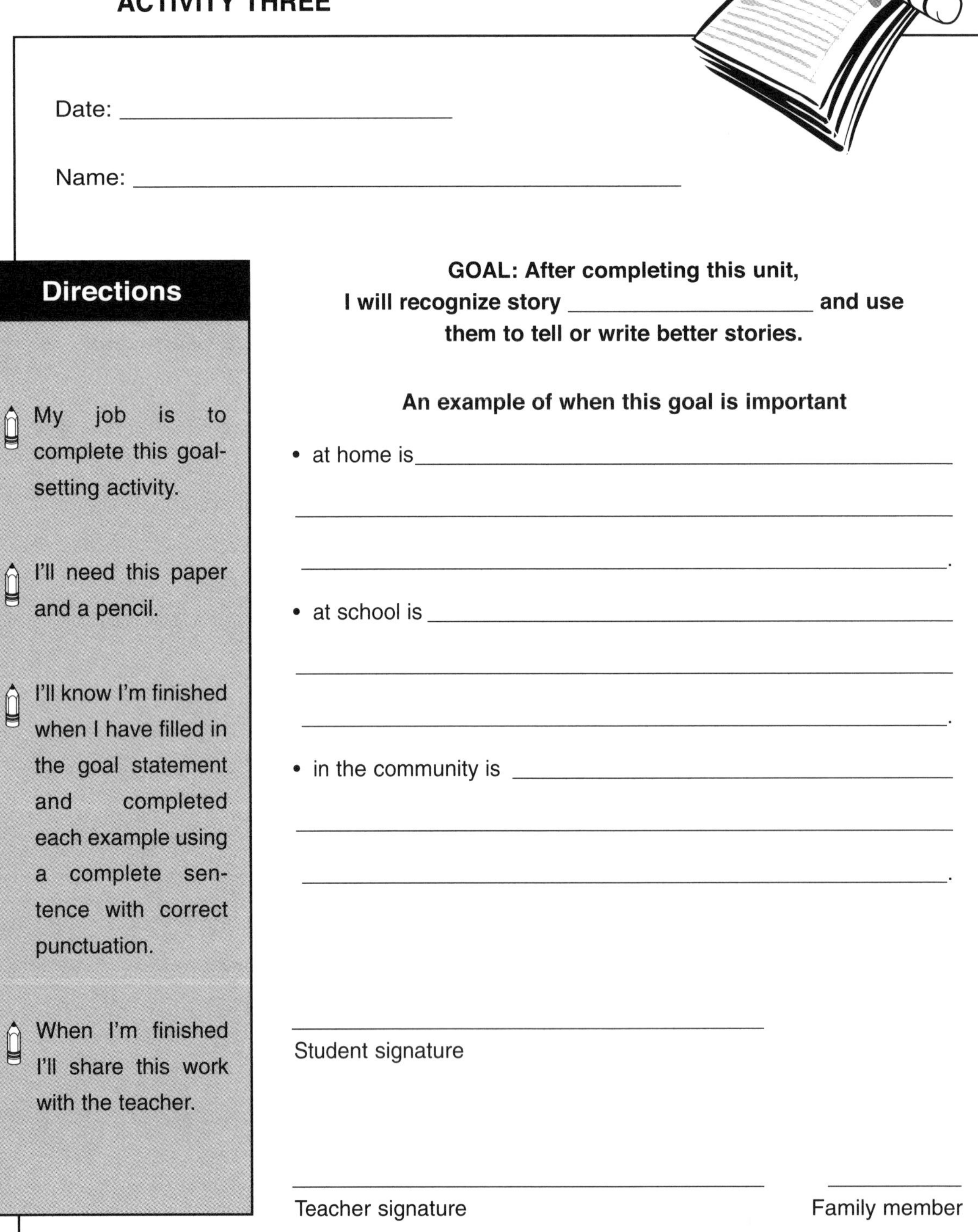

Date: ____________________________

Name: ____

Directions

- My job is to complete this goal-setting activity.
- I'll need this paper and a pencil.
- I'll know I'm finished when I have filled in the goal statement and completed each example using a complete sentence with correct punctuation.
- When I'm finished I'll share this work with the teacher.

GOAL: After completing this unit, I will recognize story ____________________ and use them to tell or write better stories.

An example of when this goal is important

- at home is ____
____
____.
- at school is ____
____
____.
- in the community is ____
____
____.

____
Student signature

____
Teacher signature

____
Family member initials

© 2001 *Thinking Publications.* Duplication permitted for educational use only.

STORY FORMULA: IDENTIFYING STORY ELEMENTS (PART I)

GOAL

To identify story grammar elements

BACKGROUND INFORMATION

The purpose of this lesson is to help students identify essential story grammar elements and use these elements to create their own stories. Before students can be expected to tell, retell, or write clear and logical stories *(Part II)*, they must be able to identify the basic story grammar elements *(Part I)*. Many variations of story grammar models exist, but the model used in this unit is based on Stein and Glenn's (1979) model and describes story grammar elements as setting (including time [when], place [where], and characters [who]), problem/event, plan and actions, and consequences/resolution.

OBJECTIVES

1. Identify story grammar elements.
2. Use higher level thinking skills to make predictions, draw conclusions, and make inferences about a story.

MATERIALS

1. *Solve the Story Formula* graphic (See page 154; duplicate and enlarge the graphic, color it, mount it onto construction paper or poster board, and laminate it for durability if desired.)
2. *Chicken Sunday* (1992) by Patricia Polacco (This book was chosen because it is easy to identify the story grammar elements. Any book with similar characteristics can be substituted.)
3. *Rapid Write: Story Formula (Part I)* (See page 155; duplicate one per student.)

INTRODUCTION

Tie-in to Prior Learning

Remind students that in *Goal-Setting Activity Three* they set a new goal. Tell students that now they are ready to begin work on the communication skills necessary to understand, enjoy, tell, and write better stories.

Focus/Relevance

Ask students if they have ever been accused of doing something that they did not do. Ask what they did to convince their accuser that they were innocent. Did students try to explain what happened or did they just get mad? Tell students that in this lesson they will listen to a story about some children who faced a similar problem.

LESSON ACTIVITIES

1. Ask students to brainstorm the elements that make up a good story. Show the *Solve the Story Formula* poster, and discuss why each of the story elements is important to the overall flow of a good story. Give examples, such as leaving out one or more of the essential elements in a chemical formula or trying to tell about a favorite movie and forgetting to mention the main character. Emphasize that the elements for a good story are just as important as the elements in a chemical formula.

2. Before reading the story, show students the cover of *Chicken Sunday* and discuss the author. Ask students to predict what they think the story might be about by looking at the front cover and title. Ask if anyone has a prediction about what kind of trouble these children might be facing in the story.

3. Tell students to listen for the story elements as you read. Ask students to signal when they recognize an element. Refer to the *Solve the Story Formula* poster as students identify each of the story elements. Read the story. Highlight the following literary components:

   - Vocabulary—*gramma/Babushka/bubbie* (various terms for "grandmother"), *hoppin' john, collard greens, spoon bread, bonnet, pelted, sobbed, lump, beeswax, funnel, counter, glowered, glistened, intricate, solo, rumbles*

   - Figurative language—*slow thunder and sweet rain, flat as a hen's tongue, old country, homeland, chutzpah, warm smile, hearts sank, hearts would burst, hearts sang*

4. When finished reading, ask the following questions:

   - How does the author let us know that the characters come from different backgrounds and different languages?

   - Why is the story called *Chicken Sunday?*

   - Why did Mr. Kodinski call the children brave when they returned to his shop?

   - Why do you think Mr. Kodinski gave the hat to the children instead of selling it to them?

   - How did Miss Eula feel when she unwrapped the hat?

- Do you think that the children had a good solution to their problem? How would you have solved the problem?

5. Review the story grammar elements in the story by referring to the *Solve the Story Formula* poster. Hand out *Rapid Write: Story Formula (Part I)*. Read through the directions as a group and check for understanding. Ask students to write a complete sentence to identify each of the story elements in *Chicken Sunday*. Remind students to reread for clarity before asking for help or finishing their work. Discuss their responses.

CLOSURE

Summarize the lesson, review its relevance to students, and tie it to future learning. Remind students that being able to recognize and use story elements is useful in both understanding stories and when telling and writing their own stories. Tell students that in the next lesson *(Story Formula: Identifying Story Elements [Part II])* they will be practicing their writing and thinking skills as they create their own stories.

Solve the
Story Formula
Setting
(Who)
(When)
(Where)
Problem
or
Event
Plan
and
Actions
Consequences
and
Resolution
Complete
Story
All these "elements" complete the story formula!

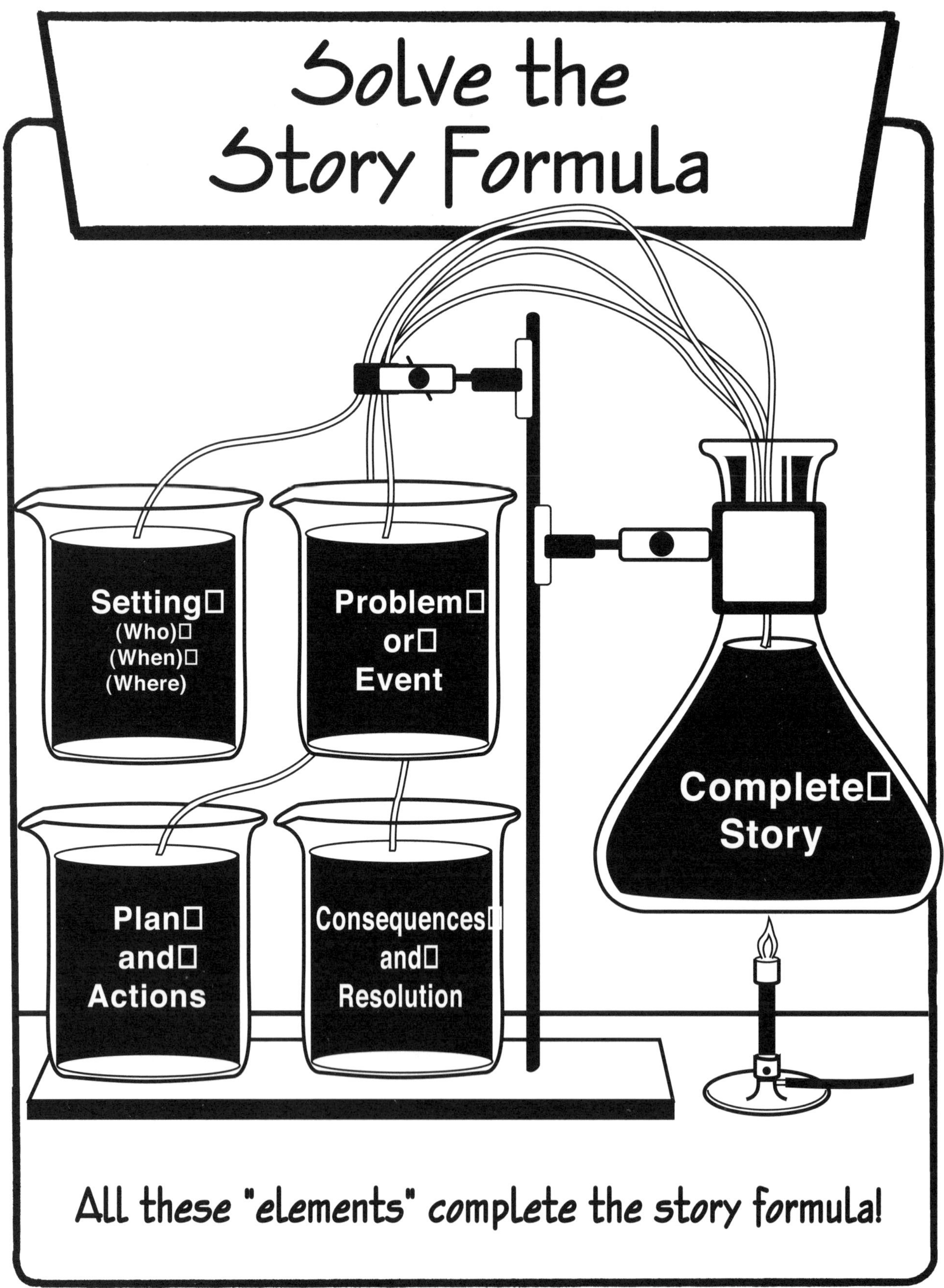

© 2001 *Thinking Publications.* Duplication permitted for educational use only.

Rapid Write

STORY FORMULA (PART I)

Date: ______________________________

Name: ____

Directions

- My job is to identify the story elements in the story.
- I'll need this paper and a pencil.
- I'll know I'm finished when I have a complete sentence identifying each story element.
- When I'm finished I'll share this work with the teacher.

Write the story elements for the story read in class.

Setting:

Time ____

____

Place ____

____

Characters ____

____

Problem or Event: ____

____

Plan and Actions: ____

____

Consequences and Resolution: ____

____

____

© 2001 *Thinking Publications.* Duplication permitted for educational use only.

STORY FORMULA: IDENTIFYING STORY ELEMENTS (PART II)

GOAL

To use story grammar elements

BACKGROUND INFORMATION

The purpose of this lesson is to improve students' overall oral and written narrative language skills. Students continue to identify story grammar elements and then use the elements to create their own stories. In *Part I,* students learned to identify basic story grammar elements, which is a skill that precedes telling and writing their own stories *(Part II).* Many variations of story grammar models exist, but the model used in this unit describes story grammar elements as setting (including time [when], place [where], and characters [who]), problem or event, plan and actions, and consequences and resolution.

OBJECTIVES

1. Identify story grammar elements.
2. Use higher level thinking skills to make predictions, draw conclusions, and make inferences about a story.

MATERIALS

1. *Solve the Story Formula* poster (Created earlier)
2. *Chicken Sunday* (1992) by Patricia Polacco (This the lesson evolves around the book *Chicken Sunday* (1992) by Patricia Polacco. If you used a different story in *Part I,* you will need to adapt this lesson.)
3. *Rapid Write: Story Formula (Part II)* (See page 158; duplicate one per student.)

INTRODUCTION

Tie-in to Prior Learning

Refer students to the *Solve the Story Formula* poster, and review the essential story elements. Let students give an example of each of the story elements from *Chicken Sunday.* Tell students that in this lesson they will be creating their own stories.

Focus/Relevance

Refer back to the problem and actions from *Chicken Sunday.* Ask if anyone has another idea about how the children could have solved their problem. Use students' suggestions to change the direction of the story, and review how a few changes can make a huge difference in the story (e.g., lead to a different resolution). Tell students that they will have an opportunity to create their own unique story by writing a plan and action as well as a consequence and resolution to a story starter idea.

LESSON ACTIVITY

1. Hand out the *Rapid Write: Story Formula (Part II).* Read the directions as a group and check for understanding. Tell students that they are given a story starter, which includes the setting and problem or event for a new story. They will have to finish the story by writing a plan and actions as well as consequences and a resolution.

2. Read the story starter together as a group. If necessary, brainstorm ideas together. Then have students write their ideas on their *Rapid Write* forms. Remind students to reread for clarity before asking for help or finishing their work. Have students share their stories as time allows.

CLOSURE

Summarize the lesson, review its relevance to students, and tie it to future learning. Remind students that being able to recognize and use the story formula is useful in both understanding stories and telling or writing stories. Congratulate students on their creative writing ideas. Tell students that in the next lesson *(Main Idea: Summarizing the Big Picture)* they will be using their knowledge of the story formula to discover the big picture of a story or article.

Rapid Write

STORY FORMULA (PART II)

Date: ______________________________

Name: ______________________________

Directions

- My job is to write the plan and actions as well as consequences and a resolution for a story.
- I'll need this paper and a pencil.
- I'll know I'm finished when I have written a plan, actions, consequences, and a resolution for the story starter.
- After I'm finished I'll share this work with the teacher.

Finish this story starter.

One crisp, cool December day a group of friends were helping their teacher decorate for a winter holiday program. They had nearly finished when class was dismissed. When they returned the next day, they found that their scenery had been ruined! Someone had drawn all over it! Parts of it were torn into pieces!

What happened next (plan and actions)? ______________________________

____

____

____

____

How will the story end (consequences and resolution)? ______________________________

____

____

____

____

© 2001 *Thinking Publications.* Duplication permitted for educational use only.

MAIN IDEA: SUMMARIZING THE BIG PICTURE

GOAL

To identify details and the main idea

BACKGROUND INFORMATION

The purpose of this lesson is to apply knowledge of story grammar elements to formulate a story's main idea and to summarize how details within a story have a common thread. This requires higher level thinking skills and offers students an opportunity to practice summarizing in their own words. Students learn that many forms of writing have story grammar elements. Information within a story may also be implied, which requires students to synthesize information not explicitly explained. This lesson may take several sessions to complete.

OBJECTIVES

1. Draw conclusions about which details in an article are significant.
2. Recognize how details within an article are connected.
3. Summarize the main idea of an article.

MATERIALS

1. *Main Idea: The Big Picture* graphic (See page 162; duplicate and enlarge the graphic, color it, mount it onto poster board or construction paper, and laminate it for durability if desired.)
2. *Pets Need Vet*s article (See pages 163–164; duplicate one per student.)
3. *Puzzle Page* (See page 165; enlarge the graphic, mount it onto poster board or construction paper and laminate it, or create one overhead transparency; also duplicate one per student.)
4. *Rapid Write: Main Idea* (See page 166; duplicate one per student.)

INTRODUCTION

Tie-in to Prior Learning

Remind students that in the last lesson *(Story Formula: Identifying Story Elements [Part II])* they practiced adding a plan and actions as well as consequences and a resolution to a story. Tell students that in this lesson they will be using their knowledge of a story formula in a different way.

Focus/Relevance

1. Ask students if they know how to identify the main idea of a story or movie. Ask why movie reviews or book reviews want to tell only a short summary of the story line. Elicit the idea that reviewers do not want to tell too many details, because that might ruin the story for others. Read the following movie summary for *Stuart Little:*

   This enchanting remake of E. B. White's classic story tells about a little mouse who was adopted by a family not as a pet but as another child.

   Ask students what they know about the movie from this short review (e.g., the characters and the potential problems). Tell students that a good summary provides enough information—the main idea—to get you interested without telling all of the story.

2. Explain that just as movie reviewers pick out key parts of an entire movie that will make the viewer want to see it, newspaper columnists and reporters have to choose important details from real-life events and use headlines that will catch readers' attention. Tell students that in this lesson they will learn a strategy for determining the main idea of an article and learn how to give a summary.

LESSON ACTIVITIES

1. Show students the *Main Idea: The Big Picture* poster. Ask students to describe what they see (i.e., the puzzle pieces). Discuss the task of putting a puzzle with many tiny pieces together. Point out that the pieces do not look like much individually but when put together make "the big picture." Ask if students or their parents read newspapers or listen to news programs. Explain that by learning to summarize what they read or hear parents can also relate the big picture to friends without giving every detail.

2. Explain to students that you will be reading them an article and their job is to listen for four details. Do not tell them the title of the article. Tell them that the author is a doctor. Have students make predictions as to what the article could be about. Do not tell them that the doctor is a veterinarian; let the realization come as they listen. Read *Pets Need Vets.* After reading, have students share four details that they learned in the article. Write each detail on one puzzle piece of the *Puzzle Page* using the transparency or the laminated poster board you created. Discuss what the details have in common. Have a student give one title for the article after discussing the common thread among the details.

3. Hand out *Rapid Write: Main Idea* and *Puzzle Page* to each student. Read the *Rapid Write* article aloud for students. Read the directions as a group and check for understanding. Tell students that they will get to practice deciding the main idea of this article on their own by finding the important details and writing them on the puzzle pieces. Have students write a title that will tie the pieces into one big picture (i.e., the main idea). Remind students to reread for clarity before asking for help or finishing their work. Let students share their summaries.

CLOSURE

Summarize the lesson, review its relevance to students, and tie it to future learning. Congratulate students on demonstrating an important skill that they will use both at school and at home. They will use this skill of determining the main idea with their friends when summarizing "cool" articles they have read or in school when summarizing chapters in books, which will help them when they are taking a test. Tell students that in the next lesson *(The Detail Trail: Linking Cause and Effect)* they will be using the details in a story to discover why different events happened—they will learn about cause and effect.

Main Idea: The Big Picture

- **Listen or read for details.**
- **Think about how details are alike.**
- **Write a title that summarizes details.**

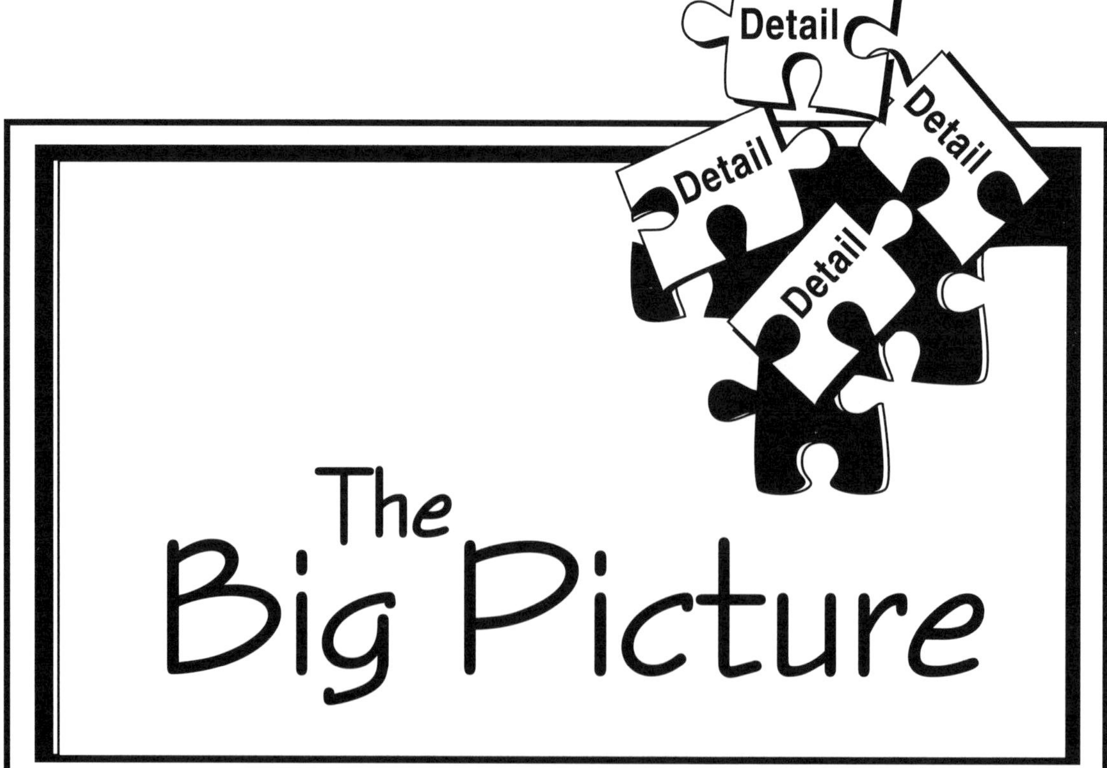

The Title = The Main Idea

© 2001 *Thinking Publications.* Duplication permitted for educational use only.

Pets Need Vets

Did you know?

Did you know that a veterinarian could be one of your pet's best friends, next to you of course? It's important to start your pet on the road to good health right from the start by scheduling a visit with a veterinarian. Ask a friend or neighbor who has pets or call the local humane society to find out the names of vets in your area.

A veterinarian checks your pet for many different things. A vet can recommend the appropriate food for your pet and the vaccinations or shots it needs. If your pet is sick, a vet can prescribe medicine. It is important to use prescription medicine from the vet rather than medicine that you purchase at a pet store. Medicines and home remedies designed for humans could be deadly for a pet.

Shots

Just like children need to receive shots to keep them safe from certain illnesses, dogs need a variety of shots to keep them healthy and safe from diseases. Dogs should receive a yearly rabies shot, and they should always wear a city or county rabies tag to show when the vaccination was given. All dogs should be protected against *distemper.* Distemper is a serious disease in dogs that causes fever, coughing, red eyes, convulsions, pneumonia, and even death. Another vaccination that a veterinarian may prescribe protects dogs from *canine hepatitis.* Vets are now encouraging pet owners to vaccinate their dogs against *kennel cough.* This illness is highly contagious and can be contracted when dogs are boarded at a kennel with other dogs.

Cats also need to be vaccinated against a variety of illnesses. Just like dogs, cats need an annual shot to prevent rabies, especially if they spend any time outdoors. Just like dogs, one of the most serious and widespread diseases for cats is called *feline distemper.* Some of the symptoms of this disease include listlessness, loss of appetite, high fever, and vomiting. Cats of all ages need to be protected from feline distemper with an annual vaccination. A veterinarian may also prescribe vaccines to prevent influenza, pneumonia, and other illnesses.

© 2001 *Thinking Publications.* Duplication permitted for educational use only.

Ear Mites

Veterinarians know that many pets may share a common problem. One of the most common and troublesome problems for cats is ear mites. If a vet notices brown material in a cat's ear, frequent head shaking, and intense scratching behind an ear, he or she will suspect that the cat has been infected by these microscopic creatures. If you notice any of these symptoms, the cat should be taken to a vet at once.

When You Should Visit a Vet

A responsible pet owner should take his or her pet to a veterinarian whenever the animal appears sick. Dogs and cats should have a regularly scheduled checkup, just like humans. Visiting a vet on a regular basis can help your pet live a longer, healthier life by catching illnesses or conditions before they become a serious threat.

Health Checklist

The following health checklist can help you stay up-to-date with your pet's health, so you know when it's time to schedule your next visit with a veterinarian.

Treatment	Date Due
1. Checkup	
2. Vaccinations	
3. Exam for ear mites	

It is also beneficial to give the vet a list of all vitamins and medications that your pet takes. Make sure that you know when the medication was started and how many times a day it is given.

© 2001 *Thinking Publications.* Duplication permitted for educational use only.

PUZZLE PAGE

Title:

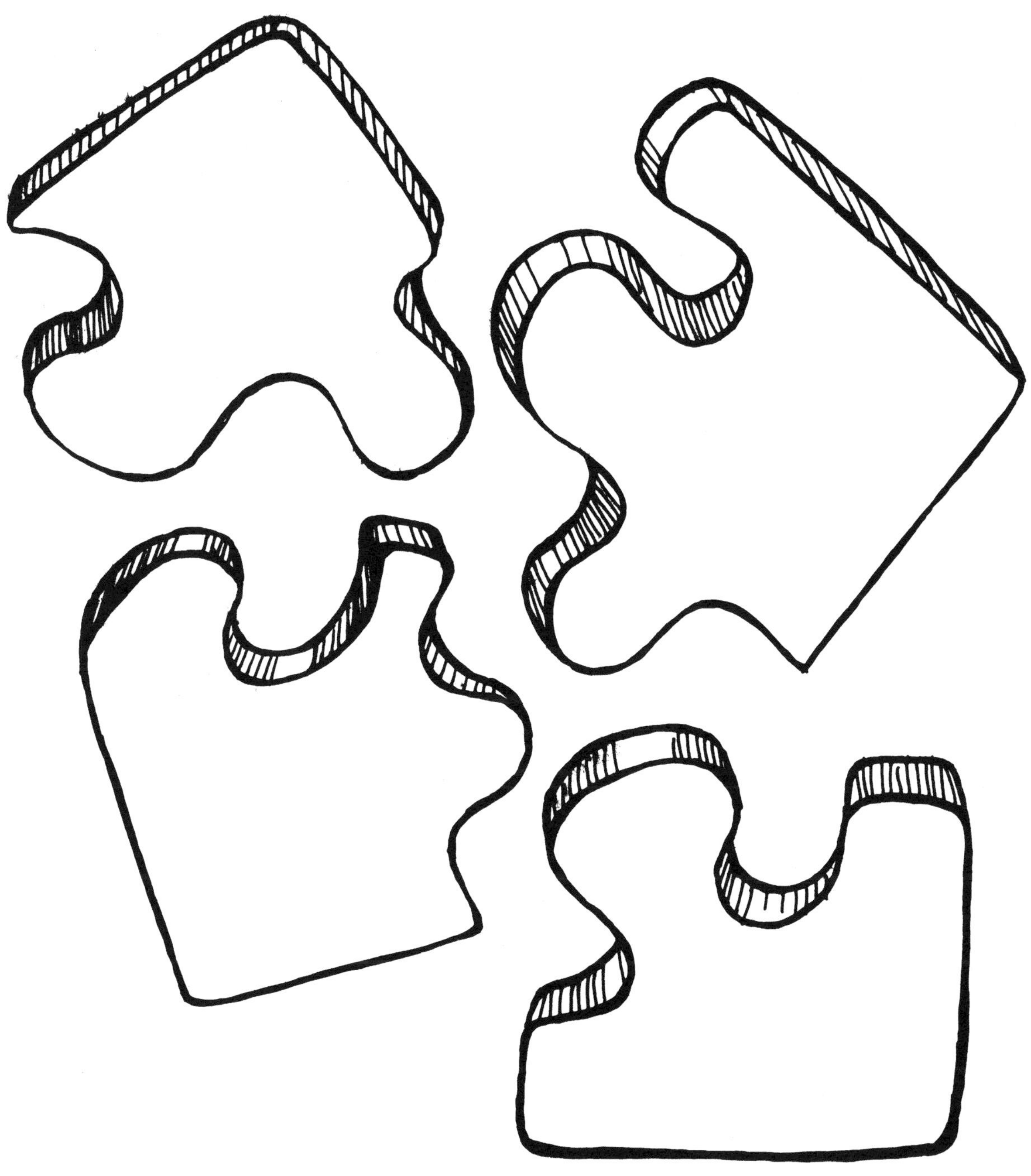

© 2001 *Thinking Publications.* Duplication permitted for educational use only.

Rapid Write

MAIN IDEA

Date: ______________________________

Name: ____

Directions

- My job is to determine the main idea of the article.
- I'll need this paper, the *Puzzle Page*, and a pencil.
- I'll know I'm finished when I have
  - read the article
  - written a detail on each puzzle piece on the *Puzzle Page*
  - decided how the puzzle pieces go together
  - written a title on the *Puzzle Page* that tells the main idea
- When I'm finished I'll share this work with the teacher.

Determine the main idea of this article.

Do you enjoy a good magic trick? If you've ever seen a magician saw a person in half or make an elephant disappear, you may have wondered how the trick was done. But would you still be amazed if you discovered the magician's trick?

Probably not! Once you know how a trick is done, the mystery vanishes. If a magician shares all his or her secrets, there is no longer any mystery and that's what keeps an audience interested. That's why magicians keep their tricks confidential.

Magic is fun for the audience because they don't know how the trick is performed. For a magician, the fun is fooling the audience with a well-performed trick.

An important rule to live by, even for an amateur, is to never reveal a trick. Even though people often ask a magician how a particular trick is done, deep down inside they really don't want to know. Don't even tell friends! Even friends aren't impressed when they learn how easily they've been fooled. The magician might want to answer the "How did you do that?" question with a clever response, such as "Quickly!" or "I thought I did it pretty well, don't you?"

Another rule of thumb is to avoid showing a trick more than once to the same audience. Since they know the ending to the trick, they may be looking for the key to your sleight of hand. Remember, most people want to believe the magic!

© 2001 *Thinking Publications.* Duplication permitted for educational use only.

THE DETAIL TRAIL: LINKING CAUSE AND EFFECT

GOAL

To recognize cause and effect relationships

BACKGROUND INFORMATION

The purpose of this lesson is to increase students' overall knowledge of story structure by helping them identify cause and effect relationships within a story context. Students will be identifying, answering, and asking questions to discover cause and effect relationships and will identify keywords that signal cause and effect. In addition, students will practice identifying complete versus incomplete thoughts using conjunctions and improve language flexibility by rearranging clauses within a sentence. This lesson may take several sessions to complete.

NOTE: The word *then* is technically a conjunctive adverb (i.e., a word that connects two sentences and provides adverbial emphasis). However, this detail is not important for students at this age level. The word *then* was included because it signals cause and effect.

OBJECTIVES

1. Understand and use the following terms: *cause, effect, clause,* and *conjunctions.*
2. Identify cause and effect relationships within a story.
3. Identify conjunctions that signal cause and effect relationships.
4. Recognize complete and incomplete thoughts that include clause words.
5. Use conjunctions to connect ideas in complete sentences.

MATERIALS

1. *Cause and Effect: Follow the Detail Trail* graphic (See page 172; duplicate and enlarge the graphic, color it, mount it onto poster board or construction paper, and laminate it for durability if desired.)
2. Strips of paper cut 11" × 4¼"
3. *Stickeen: John Muir and the Brave Little Dog* (1998) by John Muir, as retold by Donnell Rubay (This book was selected because of its interesting subject matter and the variety of cause and effect relationships depicted. Any book with similar characteristics can be substituted.)
4. *Clause Paws Cards* (See pages 173–174; duplicate one set per student onto heavy-stock paper.)
5. *Rapid Write: The Detail Trail* (See page 175; duplicate one per student.)

6. *Just Do It! Review Activity Five* (See page 176; duplicate one per student.)

7. Unit Three posters (Created earlier)

INTRODUCTION

Tie-in to Prior Learning

Remind students that in the last lesson *(Main Idea: Summarizing the Big Picture)* they pieced the puzzle together to get "the big picture." They used supporting details to summarize an article's main idea. Compliment them on their skill in determining details and the main idea to create a title that informed readers about the article.

Focus/Relevance

1. Ask students what would happen if a neighbor left the sprinkler running and there was a big freeze during the night. Ask why this event would have an effect on someone driving down the street or walking on the sidewalk the next morning. Tell students that if someone has ever experienced slipping on an icy sidewalk or street, they will be especially careful watching for ice the next time there is a freeze. Then ask, "Why would you be careful the next time there is a freeze?" Discuss their responses and point out that they have just illustrated a cause and effect relationship. Tell students that our lives are full of events that have a cause and an effect that help them learn.

2. Write the word *why* and the word *cause* beside it in parentheses where everyone can see them. Write the word *because* and the word *effect* beside it in parentheses where everyone can see them. Refer to the example of a cause and effect relationship by pointing out that the sprinkler running on a freezing cold night could cause the effect—a slip on the ice the next morning—and the slip on the ice could cause the effect of being careful the next time there is a freeze. Tell students that in this lesson they are going to be listening for the cause and effect of different events within a true story you will read to them.

LESSON ACTIVITIES

1. Show the *Cause and Effect: Follow the Detail Trail* poster and point out the keywords (i.e., *so, if, when, because, since,* and *then)* that are listed. Tell students that these are some of the words that signal cause and effect and are called *conjunctions*. Using the sprinkler example, share the following cause-effect statements:

- *Since* the sprinkler was left on last night, ice formed on the sidewalk.
- *If* a sidewalk is icy, *then* someone might fall and have an accident.
- I wrecked my car *because* I hit ice on the street.
- I slipped on an icy sidewalk, *so* I'll have to have my foot x-rayed.
- *When* water freezes on the sidewalk, the sidewalk becomes slippery.

2. Give each student some strips of paper. Have students write one clause from the sprinkler sentences on each piece of paper. Point out the clauses and how they are joined by conjunctions. Have students identify each of the clauses by telling whether it is a cause or an effect. Point out that each thought is a clause and not a complete sentence. It needs more information to complete the thought or idea and that information is added using the conjunctions. The strips of paper show the effect of rearranging the order of the clauses or using different conjunctions within the clauses.

3. Tell students that they are going to listen to a true story about an explorer. They will need to listen carefully to the events in the story, so they can answer questions about cause and effect. Remind students that by understanding why different events occurred within the story they will be able to follow its "detail trail." Tell students that some of the answers may come directly from the story, but some of the questions may require them to respond according to what they think is a logical answer.

4. Show the cover of *Stickeen.* Ask students what they predict the story will be about. Point out that the story is by John Muir but has been retold by Donnell Rubay. (There is information at the end of the book about John Muir, Donnell Rubay, and Christopher Canyon, the illustrator.) Read the story and highlight the following literary components:

   - Vocabulary—*canoe, glacier, whimper, journey, aloof, crevasses, chasms, tottered, fate, marooned*

   - Figurative language—[Stickeen was] *cold as a glacier,* [the dog] *acted distant, music and motion of the storm, queer noodle, pushed on, could not shake him, no more than the earth can shake the moon, meet one's fate,* [jumped over] *like a flying cloud*

5. Ask the following questions and tell students to answer them using a complete sentence. Remind students that they will need to listen for the critical information from the question to include the information in their answer. Explain that answering a question completely is especially important when writing answers. Possible basic questions include the following:

   - Why were the explorers taking this journey?
   - How did Stickeen get his name?
   - Why did Stickeen's owner think he was the perfect dog to take on the trip?

- Why would these traits (of the dog) be important when going to southeastern Alaska?
- Why did Muir make Stickeen moccasins?
- Why were Stickeen's feet bleeding?
- Why did Muir worry about jumping over the crevasses in the ice?
- Why did Muir not want to go back down the glacier the same way he had come up?

Higher level questions with inferred information include the following:

- Why did Muir think that Stickeen was an unusual or odd dog?
- Why do you think Stickeen was the first off the boat and the last to get on?
- Why do you think the dog wanted to go?
- Why do you think that Stickeen refused to go back to camp when Muir went exploring during the storm?
- Why do you think Muir compared the glacier to a "great, evil creature guarding a place no man had ever gone?"
- If you were in Muir's place on the glacier with Stickeen, how would you have solved the problem?

6. After answering the questions, have students cut apart *Clause Paws Cards*. Ask students to arrange the cards in pairs (i.e., match the numbered paws) on their desks with causes on one side and effects on the other. Have students connect the clauses using one or more *Clause Paws Cards* that include conjunctions. Explain that each resulting sentence could have more than one answer (e.g., "If the crevasses were too wide then they could not turn back" and "They could not turn back because the crevasses were too wide") and some sentences can be arranged in two ways (e.g., "They could not turn back, because the crevasses were too wide" or "Because the crevasses were too wide, they could not turn back"). Discuss the students' responses.

7. Ask students how using cause and effect clauses could improve their reading and writing skills. Elicit the idea of understanding and using complex sentences.

8. Hand out *Rapid Write: The Detail Trail*. Read through the directions as a group and check for understanding. Remind students to reread for clarity before asking for help or finishing their work. Let students share their written sentences as time allows. As an additional practice activity, have students take turns showing how the cause and effect clauses can change by rearranging them and using different conjunctions in them.

CLOSURE

Summarize the lesson, review its relevance to students, and tie it to future learning. Tell students that they have discovered a trail of information about the cause and effect of different events within a story. Knowing cause and effect relationships is helpful when reading and telling or writing a story. Congratulate the students on all their hard work!

JUST DO IT!

Hand out *Just Do It! Review Activity Five.* Explain that this is a homework activity that covers all the strategies from Unit Three. Refer to the Unit Three posters. Briefly review vocabulary from the posters. Review the directions for *Just Do It! Review Activity Five*. Set a due date for the assignment.

Cause and Effect:
Follow the Detail Trail
cause
(why something happens)
if
when
WARNING!
Use complete sentences!
so
because
since
then
effect
(the result, outcome, or impact)
Use clause words to connect the details!

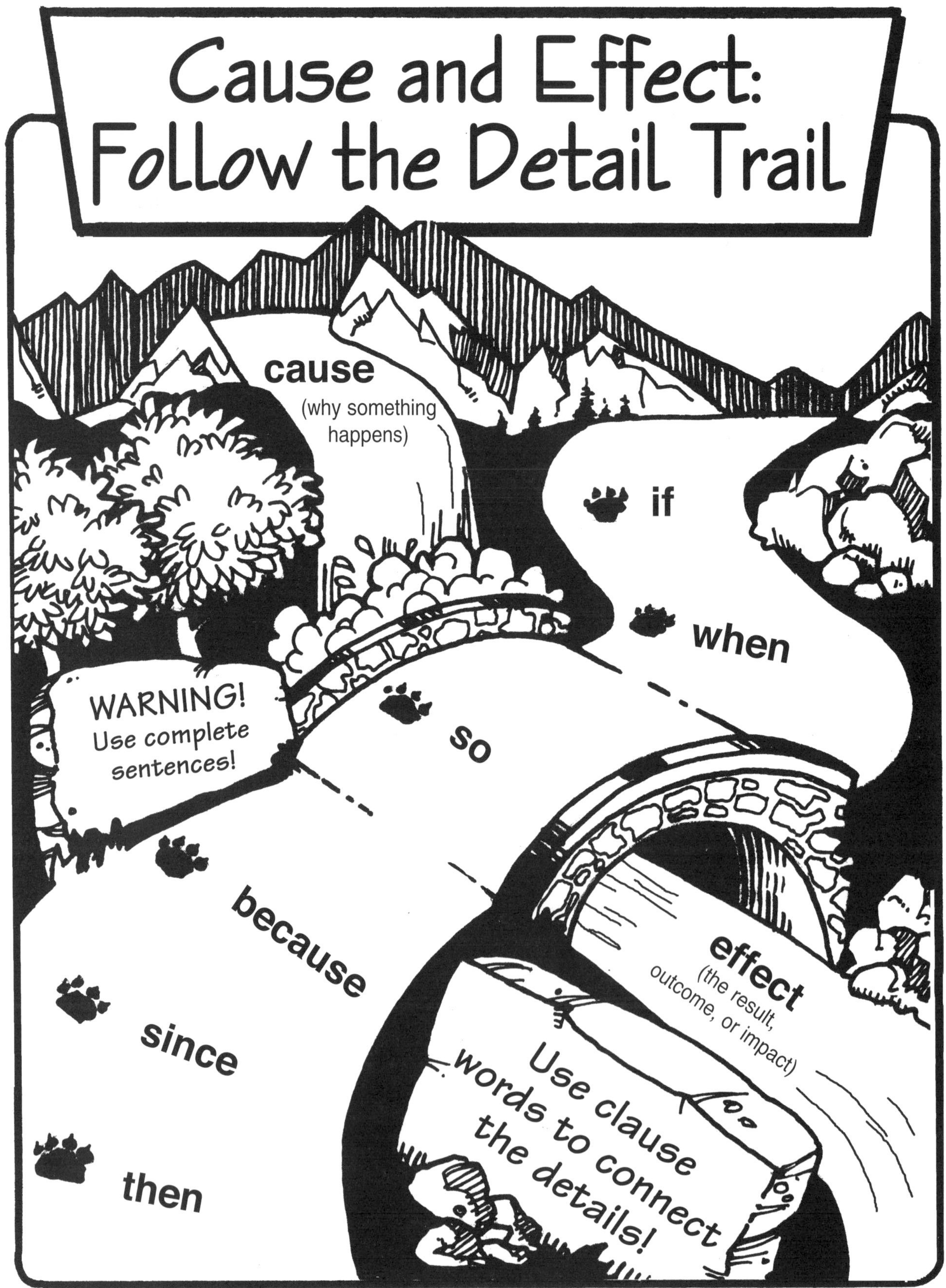

© 2001 *Thinking Publications.* Duplication permitted for educational use only.

Clause Paws Cards

the crevasses were too wide

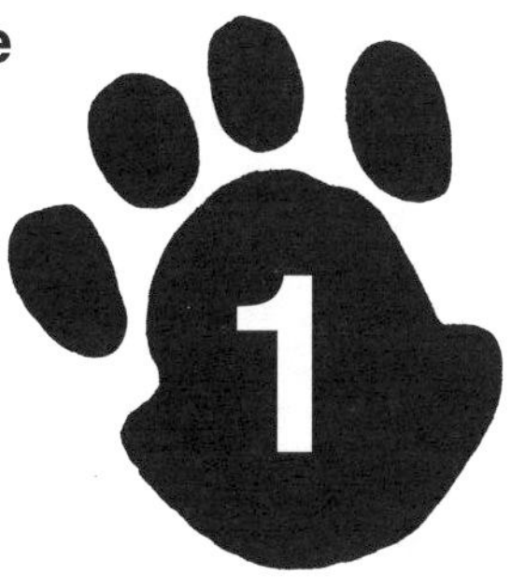

Cause

they could not turn back

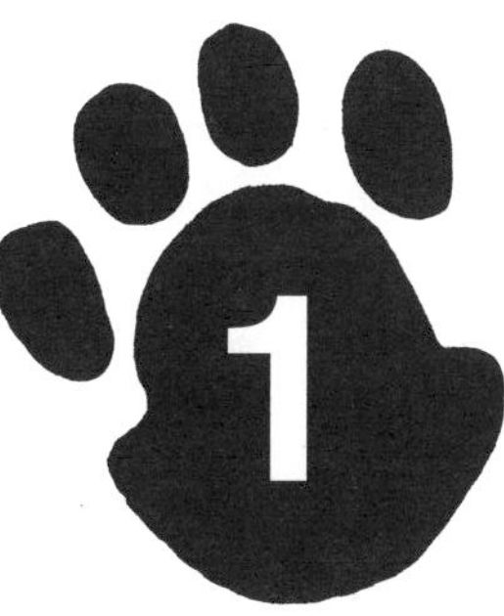

Effect

Stickeen became the explorer's friend

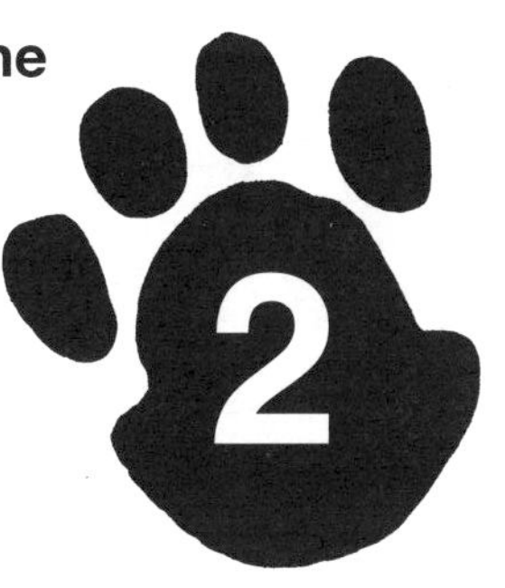

Cause

they shared a challenging and difficult adventure

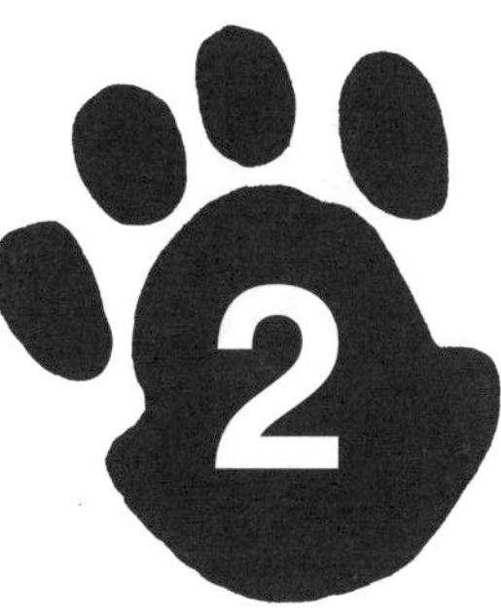

Effect

he was afraid Stickeen would be in the way

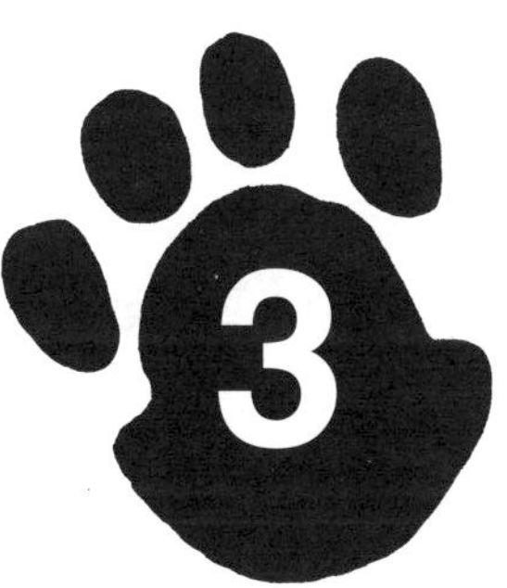

Cause

the man did not want to take the dog

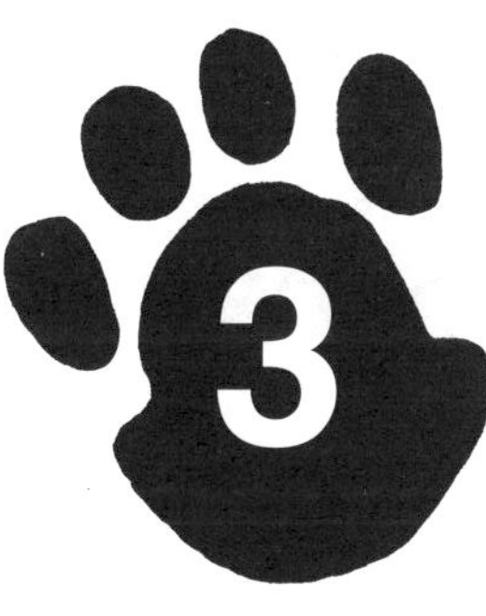

Effect

night was approaching

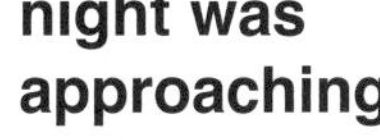

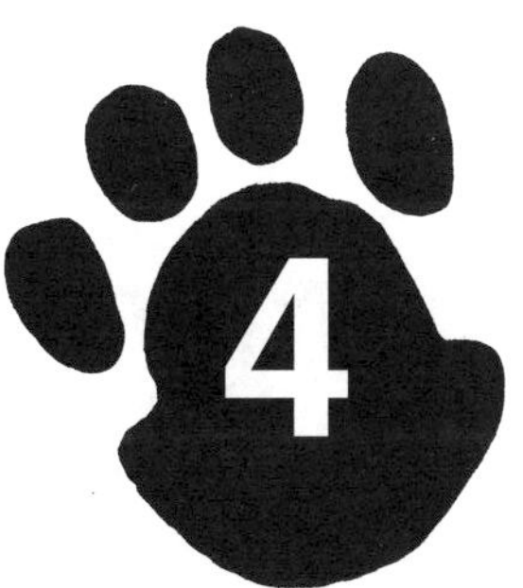

Cause

it was important to get back to camp

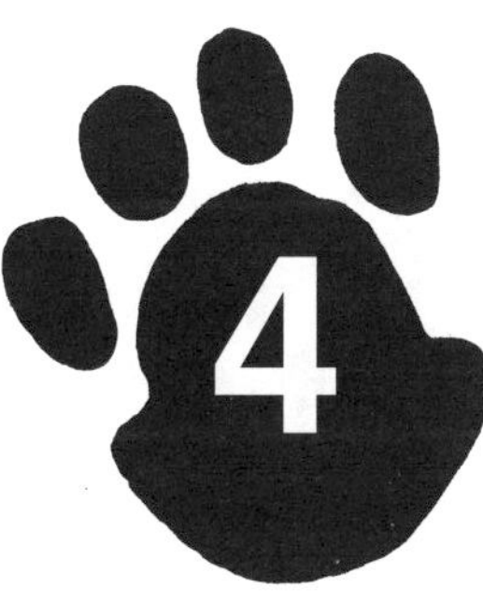

Effect

© 2001 *Thinking Publications.* Duplication permitted for educational use only.

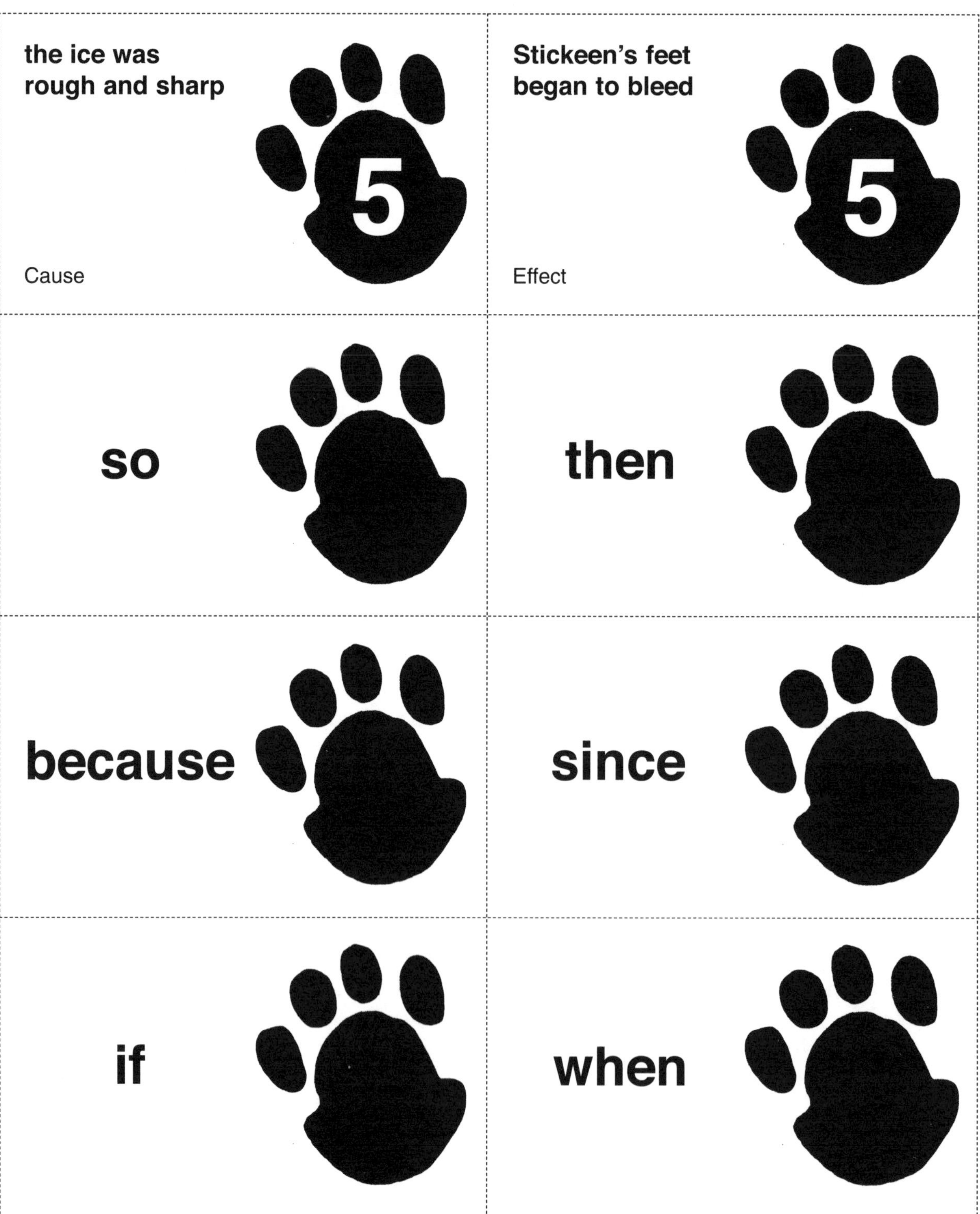

© 2001 *Thinking Publications.* Duplication permitted for educational use only.

Rapid Write

THE DETAIL TRAIL

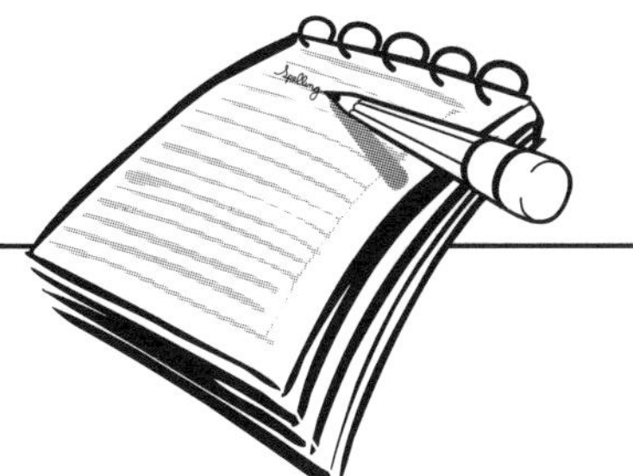

Date: ____________________

Name: ______________________________

Directions

- My job is to match the cause and effect ideas. I'll combine the ideas with a conjunction and then write them on a separate piece of paper.
- I'll need this paper, a blank sheet of paper, and a pencil.
- I'll know I'm finished when I have matched causes and effects and written 4 complete sentences on a separate sheet of paper.
- When I'm finished I'll share this work with the teacher.

Draw a line to match each cause to an effect.

CAUSE	EFFECT
I drink a lot of milk	I have a healthy heart
I do cardiovascular exercise three times a week	I have strong bones
I eat a well-balanced diet	They have a lot of vitamins and fiber in them
I eat vegetables	I will have energy to work and play

On a separate sheet of paper, use the ideas you matched above to write 4 complete sentences. Choose a conjunction from the following list to connect the ideas.

since, because, if, when, then, so

(Remember that you can arrange the cause and effect in two ways.)

© 2001 *Thinking Publications.* Duplication permitted for educational use only.

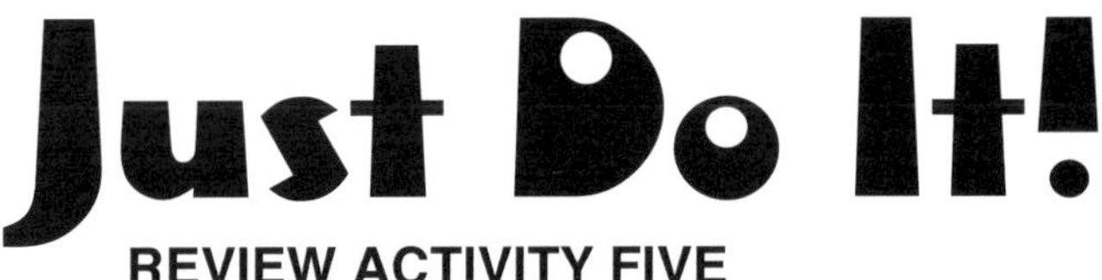

REVIEW ACTIVITY FIVE

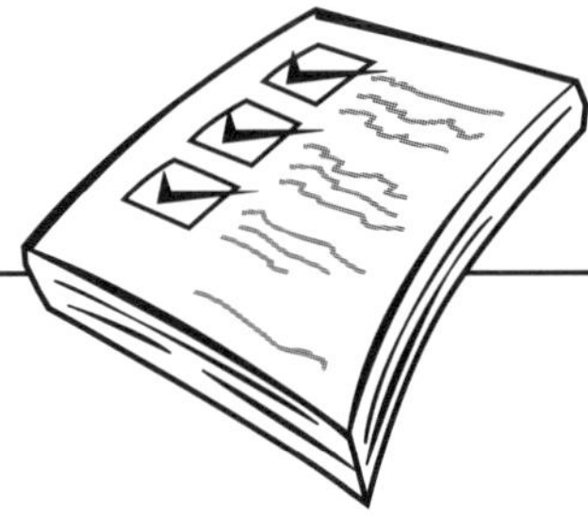

Complete the following tasks with a family member.
Initial each after you've completed it.

______ Use the story formula elements to retell a news story from T.V. or a newspaper story. Use your own words. Be sure to include the elements: setting (including time [when], place [where], and characters [who]), problem or event, plan and actions, and consequences and resolution.

______ Use the story formula elements to tell about something that happened at school today. It could be something exciting, serious, or fun.

______ Tell the main idea of a commercial you have seen on T.V.

______ Use each of the following words in a complete sentence:

then	if
when	so
since	because

This review activity is due back at school on:

Student signature ______________________________

Family member signature ______________________________

© 2001 *Thinking Publications.* Duplication permitted for educational use only.

BIBLIOGRAPHY

Baby Whale's Journey (1999) by Jonathan London
San Francisco: Chronicle Books
ISBN 0-811824-96-9

Bubba the Cowboy Prince: A Fractured Texas Tale (1997) by Helen Ketteman
New York: Scholastic
ISBN 0-590255-06-1

Chicken Sunday (1998) by Patricia Polacco
New York: Penguin Putnam Books
ISBN 0-698116-15-1

Language Strategies for Children: Keys to Classroom Success (1997) by Vicki Prouty and Michele Fagan
Eau Claire, WI: Thinking Publications
ISBN 1-888222-01-8

Language Strategies for Little Ones (1998) by Vicki Prouty and Michele Fagan
Eau Claire, WI: Thinking Publications
ISBN 1-888222-30-1

The Mary Celeste: An Unsolved Mystery from History (1999) by Jane Yolen and Heidi Elisabet Yolen Stemple
New York: Simon and Schuster
ISBN 0-689810-79-2

Rhinos Who Snowboard (1997) by Julie Mammano
San Francisco: Chronicle Books
ISBN 0-811817-15-6

See the Yak Yak (1999) by Charles Ghigna
New York: Random House
ISBN 0-679891-35-8

Stickeen: John Muir and the Brave Little Dog (1998) by John Muir, as retold by Donall Rubay
Nevada City, CA: Dawn Publications
ISBN 1-883220-78-5

Toad (1999) by Ruth Brown
New York: Penguin Putnam Books
ISBN 0-140565-50-7

Tough Cookie (1999) by David Wisniewski
New York: Lothrop, Lee, and Shepard Books
ISBN 0-688153-37-2

Turn of the Century (1998) by Ellen Jackson
Waterton, ME: Charlesbridge Publishing
ISBN 0-881063-69-X

Where the Sidewalk Ends (1974) by Shel Silverstein
New York: HarperCollins
ISBN 0-060256-68-0

REFERENCES

Bloom, B.S. (1956). *Taxonomy of educational objectives.* New York: Longman.

Caine, R., and Caine, G. (1991). *Making connections: Teaching and the human brain.* Menlo Park, CA: Innovative Learning Publications.

Chadwell, G. (1994). *Developing an effective writing program for the elementary grades.* Andover, MA: The Network.

Genishi, C. (1988). *Young children's oral language development* (Report No. PS-4-1988). Urbana, IL: ERIC Clearinghouse on Elementary and Early Childhood Education. (ERIC Document Reproduction Service No. ED 301 361)

Goodman, K. (1986). *What's whole in whole language?* Richmond Hill, Ontario: Scholastic-TAB Publications.

Hunter, M. (1982). *Mastery teaching.* El Segundo, CA: TIP Publications.

Individuals with Disabilities Education Act, 20 U.S.C. § 1400 (1997).

Johnson, D., Johnson, R., and Johnson Holubec, E. (1990). *Circles of learning* (3rd ed.), Edina, MN: Interaction Book Company.

Kavalik, S.J. (1993). ITI: *The model-integrated thematic instruction.* Los Angeles: Discovery Press.

Mesibov, G., Adams, L.W., and Klinger, L.G. (1998). *Autism: Understanding the disorder.* Norwell, MA: Kluwer Academic Publishers.

Naremore, R. (1995). *Language intervention with school-aged children: Conversation, narrative, and text.* San Diego, CA: Singular.

Oxford, R. (1994). *ERIC Digest. Language learning strategies: An update* (Report No. EDO-FL-95-02). Washington, DC: ERIC Clearinghouse on Languages and Linguistics. (ERIC Document Reproduction Service No. ED 376 707) (Available from the ERIC Document Reproduction Service, 7420 Fullerton Road, Suite 110, Springfield, VA 22153-2852)

Paul, R. (1995). *Language disorders from infancy through adolescence: Assessment and intervention.* St. Louis, MO: Mosby.

Payne, R. (1998). Learning structures. Baytown, TX: RFT Publishing.

Rief, S.F. (1993). *How to reach and teach ADD/ADHD children.* West Nyack, NY: The Center for Applied Research in Education.

Stein, N., and Glenn, C. (1979). An analysis of story comprehension in elementary school children. In R.O. Freedle (Ed.), *New directions in discourse processing* (Vol. 2 pp. 53–120). Norwood, NJ: Ablex.

Wagner, B. (1989). *ERIC Digest. Whole language: Integrating the language arts—and much more.* (Report No. EDO-CS-89-10). Bloomington, IN: ERIC Clearinghouse on Reading and Communication Skills. (ERIC Document Reproduction Service No. ED 313 675) (Available from the ERIC Document Reproduction Service, 7420 Fullerton Road, Suite 110, Springfield, VA 22153-2852)